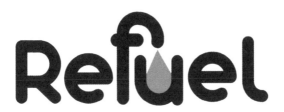

Refuel

How to balance work, life, faith and church – without burning out

KATE MIDDLETON

DARTON · LONGMAN + TODD

First published in 2015 by
Darton, Longman and Todd Ltd
1 Spencer Court
140 – 142 Wandsworth High Street
London SW18 4JJ

Illustrations in chapter 2 and chapter 9 © 2015 by Paul Rigby.

ISBN: 978-0-232-53160-2

A catalogue record for this book is available from the British Library.

Phototypeset by Kerrypress Ltd, Luton
Printed and bound by Bell & Bain, Glasgow

Contents

PART 2

How this book works

This book is written for people with busy lives, who know they experience stress and want to know how to deal with it.

The last thing you want if you are stressed is something very complicated, long or difficult to read! For this reason you'll find the book is split into manageable chapters and sections. Each one presents a topic in an approachable, easy to read way. But this book is more than just a good read – it aims to help you make some positive changes as well. So, at the end of each chapter you will find some questions which aim to help you think through what you have just read, and particularly how it applies to *your* life.

Read alone or share with a friend!

Of course this book is something you can read and ponder on your own. But it also works really well should you want to share it with other people! You can read it with a friend – and meet up to chat about each chapter. Or you can even read it as part of a small group – something more formal like a home group or group from your church, or just informally as a bunch of friends who want to get better at managing stress!

What this book isn't ...

Although this book aims to help you manage stress better, and looks at issues like burnout in more detail, it is never a replacement for proper professional support – be that from your local GP or any other healthcare professional. If you are struggling, do get advice. Should this be you, you'll find tips and suggestions to help you with this along the way.

How to read the book

This probably isn't an 'in one sitting' read. Instead I suggest that you read each chapter one at a time, setting aside time for each to ponder what you've read in more depth.

The book starts with an introduction – to fill you in a bit on where I am coming from and why I think the book is *so* important – particularly now!

Then there are two sections. The first looks in more detail at *stress* – what it is and where it often comes from. It's not just the usual old chestnuts – some of it may surprise you. I certainly hope it makes you think.

Section 2 is more practical and aims to help you think about how to make some positive changes in your life and the way you do things that might make you more effective at managing and reducing stress. You'll never get rid of it completely – but I hope that this section will help you learn how to minimise the effect it has on you.

Throughout the book there are perspectives, ideas and asides looking at stories from the Bible. I hope you'll be inspired by these – it's amazing how a book written centuries ago has so much to say to the things we are struggling with in our twenty-first-century lives. If it's not your personal faith try not to be put off or skip them – these sections are full of much wiser words than mine and they are well worth a read.

Web extras

This being the twenty-first century, we've also put together a heap of extra things you can access through the internet. Extras include links to videos, games/quizzes, relevant articles and extra information/material. Many of these will be particularly helpful if you want to work through the book as a group. Simply go to http://www.refuel1211.co.uk and enter the password REFUEL.

As part of the web extras you can also sign up to be notified when something new is added. Subscribers will also get information about relevant speaking events, conferences etc. Sign up and don't miss out!

All out for **God or** *burned out* for **God? Do** you need to *refuel?*

Stress is everywhere. At least it certainly seems to be if you read the papers. A quick scan of the headlines will usually reveal a myriad of articles about stress, containing tips to cope with stress, or often blaming stress for a bewildering list of things. But it isn't just in the papers. Ask a few people you know how they are feeling today and I guarantee that amongst the answers you will get will be either 'stressed' or 'tired'. But how concerned should we be by this? Many would say it is part of the 'buzz' of twenty-first-century life. But stress has been linked to several serious health conditions, and has been estimated to be associated with an increased risk of premature death. Might it deserve more of our attention?

What about the church?

In the midst of this stress epidemic, you might expect a message to be coming from within the church offering some kind of answer or alternative to the burnout lifestyle. But the truth is that inside the church we are just as stressed as those who are outside. Or are we? Could it be that some people inside the church are actually at *more* rather than *less* risk of stress?

As part of my job I get to travel around and speak at various conferences, training days, events, etc. Very often these are Christian events, and it is fantastic fun and a great privilege to get to meet so many people as I visit all these places. Every time after I've spoken people come to chat to me - fantastic people, inspiring people, people passionate about their faith, about God and about what they feel called to do. They are also very often people who are cracking under the weight of the stress they carry. Of course they don't always put it that way. Often they come to tell me about their struggle with their emotions - with anxiety or depression or anger. Or they might want to talk about their experiences of a particular condition - an eating disorder, or self-harm. Sometimes they come to talk about the challenges of being a leader in the church. But in all of these cases what we end up discussing is the same: how they deal (or struggle to deal) with the impact of the stress to which their lives expose them.

Work-life balance?

Stress can be a particular problem to passionate and inspired Christians. This might seem like a controversial thing to say, but in reality it is just about maths. How often have you heard people talk about the challenges of juggling work, family, and the rest of their lives? Many Christians face an additional challenge. Not only do they need to find time for their work, their family and their own lives, but also they need to fit in a couple of other things: their faith, which needs time to grow, and also makes certain demands on their time, and their church. Because on the whole, going to church is not just about going to church. Church is not a spectator sport. It is all about getting involved. I'm a leader in church and just like countless leaders across this and many other countries I have several times stood up and put all my energy and enthusiasm into hopefully igniting in the people sitting in front of me, a vision and a passion for something that requires them to give me and the church some of their time. Sometimes quite a lot of their time. For many of those people, sitting in churches across the country this and each Sunday, balancing their life is about juggling not just life and work but also their faith and the things they long to do for God and their church.

Is any of this sounding familiar to you? Have you ever had one of those moments where you try to do the maths of how you are going to fit in everything you need to do in the next few days (and preferably get some sleep at some point, not to mention hopefully manage to see some of your family within waking hours) – and realised it just isn't possible?! Have you ever got home exhausted from a bad day at work, collapsed into a chair – and then remembered you have a church meeting to go to that evening? Have you ever said yes to something at church because you know that it is something God has given you a huge passion for – something you really long to do – but then had to drop out of it not long after because you simply can't manage it on top of everything else you have to do? Have you ever fallen ill or felt dreadful and known that part of what you are feeling lies in the pace of your life in the days/weeks leading up to that point?

The problem with stress is that it takes its toll. Time and again I meet people who have been severely limited in what they can do with their lives because of the impact stress has had on them, on their families and on their mental and emotional health. So how do we manage the many demands on our time when the maths simply doesn't add up? *Should we simply be aiming to do less?*

The twin challenges

If you want to meet a guy who was all about pushing himself to the limits, Paul is a great person to start with. Reading between the lines of what he wrote, we can see a man who was incredibly passionate about what he did. Whether it was persecuting Christians or preaching to them, he threw himself 110 per cent into what he was doing. Paul was not a man who wanted to live an 'ordinary' life – he wanted to do something *extra-ordinary* with his life. He used the analogy of a race: 'Do you not know that in a race all the runners run, but only one gets the prize? Run in such a way as to get the prize' (NIV). Paul was wholehearted, focused and determined. He wanted to get the prize. In Philippians 3 he uses this analogy again: '… one thing I do: Forgetting what is behind and straining toward what is ahead, I press on toward the goal to win the prize for which God has called me' (Phil 3:13 – 14, NIV).

Paul never wanted to give any half measures – he gave everything, everything that he had. Here's an example from Acts 20, which shows how he had treated his time on mission in one area:

> You know that from day one of my arrival in Asia
> I was with you totally — laying my life on the line,
> serving the Master no matter what, putting up with
> no end of scheming by Jews who wanted to do me
> in. I didn't skimp or trim in any way. Every truth and
> encouragement that could have made a difference to you,
> you got. I taught you out in public and I taught you in
> your homes, urging Jews and Greeks alike to a radical
> life-change before God and an equally radical trust in our
> Master Jesus. (Acts 20:17–21, *The Message*).

One of Paul's main aims in life was to achieve the most he could for the thing he was passionate about: for God. It's a theme he comes back to in other letters – for example Colossians 3:23: 'Whatever you do, work at it with all your heart.' Paul's heart is clear: he wants to give it everything he has.

But at the same time Paul was aware of another vitally important aim. In Acts 20 he continues, 'What matters most to me is *to finish what God started*: the job the Master Jesus gave me of letting everyone I meet know all about this incredibly extravagant generosity of God' (Acts 20:22, 24; italics mine). Paul wasn't just about pushing himself *now* – he wanted to carry on following God and always have the energy and the passion to keep going to the end. Paul didn't just want to start the race – his aim was to *finish* the race.

In these short excerpts from Paul's farewell speech to the elders of Ephesus, he describes perfectly the twin challenges facing us as Christians. Passionate about our faith, amazed by the generosity and grace of God and inspired to share our own life-changing experience with other people, we don't want to 'skimp or trim in any way' either! We want to push ourselves to the limit to do the best we can for God. But at the same time we have another challenge: to be able to keep going. It is no use to anyone if we are only able to continue serving God for a few years and then burn out – if we start off at a sprint and soon have to stop, already exhausted. We need to be able to finish the race.

So how do we get the balance right? How do we manage this huge challenge of achieving all the things we want to, reaching for the heights that God has dreamed for us and fulfilling the potential stored within us without pushing ourselves too far? *How do we push the limits but stay sane?*

It's worth looking at how Paul managed the considerable stress he came under. Want a snapshot of Paul's stress levels? Check out his description of just some of the things he experienced in his time in ministry:

> I have worked much harder, been in prison more
> frequently, been flogged more severely, and been exposed
> to death again and again. Five times I received from the
> Jews the forty lashes minus one. Three times I was beaten
> with rods, once I was pelted with stones, three times I
> was shipwrecked, I spent a night and a day in the open
> sea, I have been constantly on the move. I have been in
> danger from rivers, in danger from bandits, in danger

from my fellow Jews, in danger from Gentiles; in danger in the city, in danger in the country, in danger at sea; and in danger from false believers. I have laboured and toiled and have often gone without sleep; I have known hunger and thirst and have often gone without food; I have been cold and naked. Besides everything else, I face daily the pressure of my concern for all the churches.
(2 Cor 11:23-28, NIV)

Paul was certainly aware of the pressure he was under and he seems to manage a key balance between his drive, and desire to achieve so much in his life and with his own realistic human limits. At the end of the day, he was able to check his ambition and drive and recognise that 'my only aim is to finish the race and complete the task the Lord Jesus has given me' (Acts 20:24, NIV). Paul knew that as big a challenge to him as the things he wanted to achieve was to make sure he kept going: to avoid burning out or dropping out, but to make it to the end.

Don't lose your zeal …

Paul was a prolific writer, with 13 New Testament books to his name. One of these is the book of Romans. Whether you think of it as a lecture or a letter, Romans is an incredible book. NT Wright describes it as 'a masterpiece' but also as 'like being swept along in a small boat on a swirling, bubbling river'.[1] As he says 'the energy and excitement of it all is unbeatable.' Written by Paul to the Christians living in Rome, it was a letter that went ahead of him as he planned to visit them, and set out some of his teachings. It is a letter full of advice, wise words, and attempts to resolve conflicts and misunderstandings that had arisen amongst this bunch of new believers.

---

1 Romans Part Two: *New Testament for Everyone*.

Romans 12 sets out Paul's key advice to live by – advice for people who are followers of Jesus in how to live their lives. This is, in essence, a summary of what Paul has learned so far on his own journey as a Christian. It is what he has learned about life. It is valuable advice coming as it does from a man who has had such an experience of God that he has turned full circle from persecuting Christians to leading them. Coming also from this high achiever, it is also advice that is particularly pertinent to those of us now, so many years later, who are living lives of trying to 'pack everything in'.

In Romans 12 Paul sets some pretty high bars for the way we live our lives – a series of do's and don'ts about how to live. Hidden amongst these is a very interesting verse for anyone struggling with stress, or wondering how to manage the various demands on their time – a verse which illustrates perfectly the tension we all carry between doing too much or doing too little. It is Romans 12:11.

How this verse is translated depends a lot on which version of the Bible you read. Here it is in the NIV: '*Never be lacking in zeal, but keep your spiritual fervour, serving the Lord.*' *The Message* translates it slightly more starkly: '*Don't burn out: keep yourself fuelled and aflame.*' However, confusingly, some other translations seem to carry completely the opposite message; here's one from the NLT: '*Never be lazy, but work hard and serve the Lord enthusiastically.*'

So which is it? Should we be taking care not to burn out, or is the message to work hard? The answer is that this verse speaks perfectly of the balance we need to manage between the two: the tension that exists in these twin challenges, to work hard and get the most out of our short time on this earth, but also to manage our energy well and make it through to the end, to avoid burnout and keep ourselves going. Too often I have heard enthusiastic preachers shout, 'I WANT TO BURN OUT FOR GOD!' To understand quite why this well-meant, passion-driven comment (more later about how passion can be related to stress) is so misguided, you need to look deeper into what Paul meant when he wrote this short but impactful verse.

To understand fully what Paul is saying, you need to look at the original language he used. At the time of writing this my family and I are living in France – a fantastic experience made all the more challenging and rich by the fact that we are living and working in a different language from our native tongue. We are experiencing daily at first hand the way in which you can lose some of the meaning of your words when you try to translate into a different language. Sometimes you can translate directly, but often – particularly when there are more complex meanings – something is lost; the essence of what you are trying to say is there, but the nuances of your message can get lost. Paul was of course writing in Greek – one of the primary languages of the Roman Empire. Greek was also one of the most 'international' languages of the time – a language spoken by a lot of people across the Roman Empire. As such it was perfect for an epistle which Paul hoped would be read by many hundreds of people – as indicated by the subscript found on many manuscripts 'for the Romans'.

The Greek word used in the key part of Romans 12:11 is *okneros*. This word can have a variety of meanings dependent on the context, ranging from to *delay/lag behind*,through to *to be slow/hesitant* or *to feel lazy/lethargic, lacking in energy* – or, as the NIV translates, 'zeal.' This is what we need to avoid – losing energy meaning that we drop back or lag behind. There is a sense of having lost the passion that drives us, the drive that keeps us going. In this context it isn't about laziness, it is about losing your energy, or running out of fuel.

In this verse, *okneros* is used in direct contrast to another word – the Greek word *zeo*. The meaning of this word is focused all around heat: to boil with heat or be aglow, aflame, hot. You can understand its meaning more clearly by looking at some other contexts in which it was used – for example in Acts 18:25, where we learn that Apollos 'had been instructed in the way of the

Lord, and he spoke with great *fervour* [*zeo*]', or in Titus 2:14: we must be a people '*eager* [*zeo*] to do what is good'.

So, to totally understand Romans 12:11 we need to think about both these meanings together. We are advised by Paul to aim to be fervent in the way we live our lives: to boil with heat; be aflame, to be energetic, 'hot' and passionate for God. Here then is the sense of pushing the limits, doing all we can to use our lives and gifts as an offering for God. However, we must make sure that while living like this we do not lose our 'zeal' – our energy, our drive and passion. *We are not called to burn out for God!* Instead we should work to the maximum of our potential but tread carefully the line between that and pushing it too far. The RSV puts it nicely: 'Never flag in zeal, be aglow with the spirit, serve the Lord' (Romans 12:11, RSV). Here lies the warning to manage our energy sensibly: to tread carefully the line between being all-out for God and burned out for God.

Don't hold back!

Paul's message in Romans 12:11 – and the message of this book therefore is *not one of holding back*. Too often the message about stress management is one that makes us feel guilty for trying to do so much in the first place. But our *zeo* is a good thing: a God-given thing, an excitement and passion, a sharing of something of the heart of God. There may be some sensible changes you need to make to your lifestyle in order to manage stress well. But good stress management isn't just about giving up the things we feel passionate about. Too many people who struggle with stress are advised to give up a lot of the things they love doing. Disempowered and demoralised they step away from jobs they love, ministries they are sure they are called to, situations, people and places they are passionate about. That is not the answer. The key to managing stress is not one of cooling down or suppressing your passion/zeal. It is as Paul advised – keep your zeal, but also keep yourself well fuelled and energised. Manage stress well, so that you stay on fire instead of burning out.

In John's gospel, Jesus makes a number of statements about who he is, trying to explain to the people around him why he was there. Probably the most well-known is in John 10:10: 'I have come that they may have life, and have it to the full' (John 10:10, NIV). There are various different translations of this verse but all have that sense of something *more* – life in a form that is bigger, better, more than the alternative without Jesus would be. The King James Version talks of having life 'more abundantly'. Perhaps my favourite translation comes from *The Message* which talks of 'real and eternal life ... more and better life than they ever dreamed of' (John 10:10, *The Message*).

It all brings to my mind the image of a swing. Not just any swing. It is a swing that was in the grounds of the primary school I went to as a child. To this day I can visualise that swing clearly, in my mind like an old sepia photograph. It had huge, tall posts that seemed to reach high into the sky, as high as the trees that stood next to it. The swing took ages to get going, so there was always a queue and if you managed to get onto it, and have time to get the best out of it before the end of playtime, you were lucky. But it was so worth it. Because once you were working that swing well, you didn't just swing – you soared. High in the air, effortlessly, wonderfully free, that swing was like no other. It was everything a swing could ever be and more.

When I read John 10:10, I think of that swing, but also of other swings I have seen – the ones I came across once with my daughter when she was young which had chains on them only a few feet long, so no matter how hard I pushed, she never really got any kind of swing worth having. Or the ones in our local village playground when I was a teenager, swings which would have been great except someone had spun them over and over the bar until they swung high out of reach on tiny chains. You can still swing on these swings, but it isn't the same. You can't get going. You can't sweep through the sky, or experience the true joy they were designed to provide. Too many people live life like this, limited, shortened by stress or the impact of stress on their lives. God does not call you to live a half-life. God wants more for you – better than you could ever have dreamed of.

Jesus came so that we could have life in all its fullness – life where we soar. His wish for us all is that through Him we can reach our full potential and *really* experience life. Life to the full is life lived to the max, life where we squeeze every last drop out of it. It is life where we achieve the most we can and truly reach our potential. This is life where we soar. It is not a life of doing less.

The most important thing you do …

So, I wonder how you are feeling as you are reading this. Full of energy? Worn out? Or just flagging a bit? The truth is that if you want to get the most out of your life – if you want to soar – learning to manage stress well is likely to be the most important thing you do. I see and get to talk to plenty of people who are unlikely ever to be limited in what they achieve in life by their ability. They are very able and very talented in their fields. Neither will they be limited by any lack of passion or drive. They are well motivated and highly driven to go the extra mile and achieve the best they possibly can. No, the reality is that many of them are being limited by the impact of stress, and by the fact that at no point have they ever learned how to deal with stress healthily. In the twin challenges of life they run well, but there's a very real risk they won't make the finish line at all. Instead they are forced to leave careers and causes they are passionate about. They wrestle with the clash between a heart which is passionate for a cause, and a body and mind which seems unable to deal with the challenge of going for it.

If you want to push the limits in your life – if you want to achieve the most you can for God, the most important thing you may ever do is take the time out to work through the things covered in this book. If, like Paul, you want to run to win the race, make sure you learn how to sustain your energy – your zeal – right through to the end. Learn what to do in those times when life seems to go crazy. Learn how to recuperate when your energy levels are being drained on every side. Learn the rhythms you need to set into your life in order to make sure you are refuelling your energy regularly. Stay energised, stay healthy, stay *'fuelled and aflame'* (Romans 12:11, *The Message*).

PART I

I

I'm *stressed*, get me out of here!

The first step on our journey to learn to manage stress is to spend some time thinking about what exactly we mean and understand by the word. 'Stress' is a word that is used a lot. But what do we actually mean? And how does this correspond to the way stress *really* affects us?

Does stress always = dis-stress?

Very often the way we use the word 'stress' gives us away. Many of us carry round a basic misconception about what stress really is. Think about the last few times you heard someone mention stress. Chances are that they were saying something like 'I'm totally stressed today'; 'She's so stressed out'; 'Don't stress, I'll do it!'; etc. Most people use the word 'stress' to describe an emotional state. So, if someone is 'stressed out' it generally implies that they are anxious, tightly strung, perhaps prone to losing their temper. When your teenager tells you to 'Stop stressing' s/he means that s/he feels you are getting wound up emotionally over something when there is no need.

There's another implication in the way we use the word stress. Being stressed is often seen as a negative thing - a sign of some kind of weakness or a good reason to avoid someone. So you might hear, 'Steer clear of her today, she's stressed out', or, 'Take no notice, he's just having a stressy day.' Being stressed implies someone who is in a very emotional state, and perhaps not as in control as they would ideally be. Someone who is regularly prone to stress problems therefore is often implied to have some kind of weakness - and there's often a sense of failure as well: 'He couldn't take the stress.'

The truth about stress

The truth about stress is a long way from the way we tend to talk about it, and it's good to remind ourselves of this. In biological terms, stress is how we describe what happens when our circumstances or situation change, and we need to adjust. Therefore, *stress describes any change which requires us to respond.*

Using this literal definition therefore, you could say that you are under 'stress' from the moment your alarm goes off in the morning. The fact that it is now morning means there are several things going on which require you to adjust and respond. You have woken up - literally you have become conscious (aware) of your surroundings, and your brain is being bombarded with signals. Most of all, it needs you to become more alert - and quickly - so you can start interacting with your environment. And there will be a host of goals you need to achieve which immediately hit the top of your awareness as you start to get on with your day.

Your body has at its disposal a whole system - a complex combination of nerves, hormones and other chemicals - which enable it to respond to the demands of your environment and the goals you need to achieve. Called the 'autonomic' nervous system, it's not something we're consciously aware of and it usually works pretty much on its own. It has two halves -

the first, the sympathetic system, is the one that controls what we classically refer to when we talk about the stress response (often called the 'fight or flight response – more about this in a moment) whilst the other, the 'parasympathetic' system, deals with what you might call the 'housekeeping' things like digestion, temperature balance, etc. (sometimes referred to as the 'rest and digest' system!). The two systems work together – when one is turned *up* the other turns *down*. That's one of the reasons why you often feel drowsy after a big meal – your body is asking you to doze, so the sympathetic system can turn down leaving the parasympathetic free to deal with all that food.

When we're talking about stress, it's the sympathetic nervous system we're interested in. From the moment you wake up, it starts to control your ability to respond to whatever the day throws at you.

Fight or flight

The sympathetic nervous system is a very complex one, with links throughout your body. Stress therefore, is much more than 'in your head' or 'just' emotions – it is about very real physical and physiological changes triggered by this system.

However, stress often does involve emotions – especially those linked to fear and anger. Emotions are used by your brain to signal and warn of changes or circumstances going on around you which might be significant or important to you, or goals you care about. So, if you walk out into the road and fail to notice a bus coming straight at you, your brain will trigger an emotion – anxiety – to alert you to this. The first and perhaps most important element of this emotion is mediated by your sympathetic nervous system, releasing a rush of adrenaline into your blood stream. This triggers physiological changes which you will almost immediately become aware of as your heart races – the classic 'fight or flight' response.

The fight or flight system mediates a whole host of responses which are designed to prepare you for action. Imagine that you are walking down the street one day and suddenly someone comes up behind you and claps their hand onto your shoulder. Assuming this was unexpected, you will feel the rush of adrenaline almost instantly: in a split second your heart will start beating faster, you will feel yourself tighten up and your breathing will speed up as well. At the same time other changes will be going on which you are probably less aware of. Blood is immediately diverted away from your digestive system and towards the major muscles of your body; the level of glucose in your blood rises and so does your blood pressure – all these changes are designed to give your muscles what they need in case they have to put in some serious work – to run away or to fight for your life.

'Chronic'/longer term stress

These kind of 'acute' (short term) challenges are fairly easy to identify – they represent immediate and occasionally dramatic challenges to us. They are short-term examples of the stress system in action. But stress can affect us in a number of other ways as well, particularly when a challenge or concern has a longer duration. It might be something subtle – a low-level anxiety/worry or the need to focus attention on something. Or it could be a longer term change – something which requires you to concentrate over a long period of time, or to be 'on alert' for a sustained period of time.

For these more long-term stressors, it is a group of hormones called glucocorticoids that become more significant. Of these, the most well-known is called Cortisol. Cortisol release is triggered by the sympathetic nervous system at the same time as adrenaline, but has its action slightly more slowly. So while adrenaline kicks in in a matter of seconds, cortisol (and the other glucocorticoids) have their impact over longer periods of time: minutes, hours, etc. A 'chronic' (longer term) stress response might therefore be mediated by heightened levels of glucocorticoids like cortisol in the blood, but also by frequent spikes of adrenaline as individual challenges and stresses occur. In fact, individual stresses differ in how they trigger levels of these two chemicals: adrenaline and cortisol – to such a degree that some scientists argue that specific stresses have their own physiological 'fingerprint' in terms of the response that they trigger.

Together therefore, hormones like adrenaline and cortisol enable us to respond to the whole range of stresses that may occur – from short term dramas through medium term social tensions to everyday challenges which require us to 'up our game' in terms of attention and concentration. Imagine, for example, that you need to drive from London to Edinburgh. This may feel like a pretty boring day – but for your body and brain it is going to be a busy one. The action of driving doesn't involve much physical work but it does pose a challenge to your brain, requiring you to remain alert, coordinate different systems (linking what your feet are doing with what your hands are doing, and what your eyes are seeing on the road, for example). Such heightened levels of attention are mediated by hormones like cortisol. Then there is the potential for the unexpected: on a busy road in particular your stress system is constantly on alert, keeping you ready to respond and triggering necessary responses with short bursts of adrenaline.

Our two stress problems

There are two main problems for humans where stress is concerned. The first is the incredibly complex nature of our world – particularly our social world. Imagine for a moment the life of your cat (or someone else's cat if you don't have one!). Their life is pretty simple all in all – if they're anything like mine a lot of it is spent sleeping. In the few hours a day when they are conscious, there are few triggers for their sympathetic nervous system. The odd mouse-chasing scenario, or perhaps next door's cat straying into their territory – on the whole these are fairly acute short term situations.

We, in contrast, live tremendously complicated lives. Our massively developed brains mean we have a heightened awareness of not just our own situations but those of people around us. Our complex social worlds mean that we frequently need to respond not to life and death situations, but to the needs and demands of relationships at many different levels. We also juggle a lot of demands: not just the simple ones of eating and sleeping but those of work, our families, our friends, etc. Imagine if you wrote out everything you needed to achieve in the next 24 hours. I mean *everything!* Including eating, sleeping, the people you need to see and spend time with, the things you must do for others, your work commitments, the jobs around the house, the financial tasks you have been putting off for weeks, those people you need to phone, the emails you need to respond to, your Twitter account … feeling like you need to take a few deep breaths? That's how complicated your world is. Your stress system helps you deal with all these demands. So in that moment when you are scrolling through your emails and you suddenly see one from your boss – 'Subject: Need to see you NOW!' – your sympathetic nervous system flicks into action just as it would had a bear jumped out in front of you.

The second way in which our stress experience differs from other mammals is all about one word: anticipation. As humans our minds are so active and reactive that we do not only exist in this moment – we exist in several others as well. Like the Mirror of Galadriel in Tolkien's *The Lord of the Rings*, our stress systems see many things – including those that have already happened and those which are (or may not be) yet to come. This means that in any one moment we might be responding not only to the stress of now, but also dwelling on the stresses of yesterday and worrying about the possible stresses of tomorrow. In fact we often 'work through' so many potential scenarios for the future, it is as though we experience the stress of several different futures - most of which will never actually happen.

I remember well a situation when a friend who I usually kept in fairly regular contact with suddenly vanished from my life for several days. Nothing happened - I just didn't hear from her for a while. It didn't take long for my sympathetic nervous system to kick in. I began to worry that I had offended her in some way, upset her, or forgotten something important - a birthday perhaps. After a day or so of worrying about this, and some checking to verify I hadn't forgotten anything significant, I moved on and began to feel cross. How dare she not talk to me for whatever reason it was! This was entirely inappropriate and childish behaviour on her part. I began to feel distinctly angry and think about how I would defend myself when I did next talk to her. After a while though, thankfully, my more rational side kicked in and I decided to call her. It turned out she had lost her phone and so she had been unable to text/call. Crisis resolved! But think about what happened to my stress system. All those emotions - all that stress - and all for a situation that existed only in my mind!

Stress is real

So, stress involves some very real physical changes. And it isn't 'optional' - you cannot 'switch off' your stress response, although you may well be able to mediate how often it is triggered and to what degree it (more about that later). Stress - the need to respond and adjust to the world around us - is *an inescapable part of being human*. It is not a weakness, or a sign of being flawed in some way. Some of us really need to hear this. If you are struggling with stress do not beat yourself up about it. It is probably because you are trying to be a superhuman, when really you are 'just' human.[1]

What about church life?

Bearing all this in mind, it's interesting to think for a moment about the particular qualities of life within the church. Most people would probably imagine church life to be particularly calm, benign and gentle. But is that realistic? Bearing in mind what we know about humans, could church life carry a stress risk?

The thing is to remember that although we bank on a considerable amount of divine influence, the people in the church are still human. And in fact, it could be argued that your average church brings together a group of humans who would not in other circumstances be brought together. This has been the way ever since the first church was described in Acts 2 - when a bunch of people who previously thought of themselves as very different from this group of Jesus's followers suddenly turned and referred to them as 'brothers' (Acts 2:37).

This socially complex group therefore means we can expect to need to deal with some challenges that arise in the relationships we share. It also means that making decisions or achieving goals together might involve more stress than we'd imagine - simply because of the inescapable dynamic of all of those people brought together.

There are other elements of church life, of course, which might be associated with greater stress. Consider, for example, these four widely recognised features of a stressful working environment...

---

1 Disappointed? So many people are when I break this news to them. If you are one of them, consider for a moment what that means. You may be ambitious, driven, keen to push yourself hard. But if even Jesus could not escape the limits of being human, neither can nor should you be able to.

So much to do but so little time. Stress is always greater when you have ambitious goals, and particularly so when your time to achieve those goals is limited. In church life it's not unusual to find ourselves working to achieve often very difficult goals in our 'spare' time. The vast majority of church workers are volunteers, giving time to the church alongside their 'day' job or other life demands. They find themselves coordinating teams, planning events, juggling budgets and leading others in whatever time they can find. It doesn't matter how committed you are to the goal; this sort of situation is inevitably going to generate some stress. In fact the more passionate you are, the more stressful you are likely to find it (see 'Is your passion stressing you out'). Passion also means that goalposts often shift – and goals may well expand if they are successfully met. So, 'This year's event went well – next year we'll push ourselves to do something *even bigger*'; 'We managed to feed 20 at our harvest supper – next time let's try to manage 40'; 'We did a great home group series this time – how about next time if we make booklets for everyone as well?' We want to be continually pushing ourselves, and our spirit is one of desiring growth – this drive is great and a really vital feature of a spiritually alive churches. But it also means we may need to be very good at managing stress.

High effort but low/no feedback. This is an inescapable experience and one you cannot fail to share if you work with … people! If you work in an environment where results are marked by something tangible – sales figures for example, although it is far from stress free, what is great is that you do get very clear feedback. If you are doing well therefore, you know about it – and you tend to get patted on the back either literally or metaphorically. Working with people (note – I don't mean working alongside people – I mean where the outcome of your work is measured in how people change, react and develop) is much harder than this. It is much harder to gauge how *you* are doing, because every outcome involves two variables – you and the other person! You could do everything right and things still not turn out the way you hoped. (On the other hand sometimes you don't do a great job but the other person pulls it out of the bag!) Feedback is more difficult – and often is much more 'enthusiastically' given if things are *not* going well! Feedback is also very influenced by the perspective of the person giving it – and the same event or situation can look totally different from someone else's perspective. So the feedback you get may not actually correspond with your energy expenditure, or how well you did.

Note that this feature may be a particular problem for people working 'behind the scenes'. A big event like a Christmas service may take months to arrange and plan but on the night, who tends to get the feedback? Generally those who are 'up-front'. But very often the people working hardest in our churches are those no one ever sees.

Multi-role situations. These are the kinds of scenario where you find yourself trying to wear many different 'hats' at once. So, you are at the same time a friend, a pastor and (apparently) a counsellor. Or you are required to be at the same time a parent, a church leader and the loyal best friend of the 'person who is very cross'. Trying to fulfil several roles at once can literally pull us in different directions – and it is something that can happen all the time in a church environment.

Note that these multi-role scenarios are particularly challenging when the boundaries between your different responsibilities are very vague. Sometimes the biggest issue in life isn't the roles you are expected to fulfil but the overlap between them. One of the most wonderful things about church life is the way we live together as family and share so much of our lives. But the fact is that this can sometimes trigger stress – particularly for those of us who call the same church both 'work' and 'family'. Most people, particularly those in caring professions, have very clear boundaries around the people they work with or 'treat' and their social life. But for those working/ volunteering in the church, work, family and social life tends to involve a lot of the same people.

This overlap means that you can go to an event expecting to wear one hat (or no hat at all) and then find that someone else is assuming you are there in a certain capacity. Ever spent an entire party talking about the problem with your after-service coffee system? Ever gone for a pub lunch with your family and run into someone who then spends half an hour delivering a detailed critique of your last sermon/Bible study? Or been in a situation where you're waiting to collect your child from youth group and chatting with other parents when suddenly up comes the subject of the cost of the weekend away, or the policy on whether phones are allowed, or what time the group starts and ends, or whatever is currently creating conflict? You want to take part in the chat as a parent because you, like everyone else, share some of those frustrations. But you cannot get away from the fact you also have a role as a leader in the church, and your responsibility therefore is to support difficult decisions. These kind of scenarios where our roles overlap can leave us constantly experiencing a low level of 'alert' and really challenge us about when exactly we are able to totally relax.

The other problem with these situations, particularly for people who are in a position of authority, is how hard it is to find people you can really be 'yourself' with. Your role may result in a certain dynamic with people, where you are expected – rightly or wrongly – to fulfil a certain role. This can mean that you find very few circumstances when you can let that go. Or, particularly if that dynamic is one of your role being very supportive/caring (for example for those who are leading or pastoring a church) it can be very hard to find spaces and people who support and feed you. Leadership can be a lonely place, and the more isolated you feel, the greater your stress load will be.

Feeling 'out of your depth'. It makes sense doesn't it, the more you feel capable and experienced in the role you are expected to fulfil, the less stress you feel. But what about living a life where by definition we want to push ourselves one step beyond that comfort zone? The church is an amazing place to grow and develop and there is the opportunity with God to do way beyond what we ever thought we would be capable of. But we mustn't deny the fact that this means we might need to deal with more stress. Of course, our learning curve is to get better at relying on God rather than ourselves – and accepting that it is often in our weakness that God can do the most. But most of us can remember examples of situations where we got properly stressed out because we weren't sure we were going to be any good at what was expected of us! Remember the first time you led prayers in your home group? Or that time you had to give a testimony in church? These are all great things to do – but for many of us stepping out of our comfort zones triggers something of a stress reaction.

This is particularly the case if our role suddenly becomes one of authority. So many people have loved their home group, toddler group, guys group, etc. – until they agreed to start trying to organise it. Suddenly the people who you thought were fun seem annoying, the ones who were zany and a good laugh are just plain irritating, and the fact that no one turns up until at least 15 minutes after you were supposed to start is actually quite big problem rather than just something to laugh about. When you carry authority things suddenly begin to matter more than they did before, even though actually nothing has changed except your perspective.

Do the 'hard work'!

There's a risk that this all sounds very negative – be reassured that it is not meant to be. I love the church and am a huge fan of the dynamic and testing environment it operates in. I love the way it brings people together who wouldn't normally share the same space, and I love the tension, promise and possibility that produces. Many of these things that are so common in church environments are also great signs of groups or organisations which are really alive – dynamic vibrant communities with a great mix of people. The church's main strength is in its uniqueness – in the unpredictable mix of people who end up sharing the same space, passions and events. I wouldn't work anywhere else! Our big mistake is if we think that living or working in this kind of place should be easy. James 3:17 contains some real wisdom on this matter: 'You can develop a healthy, robust community that lives right with God and enjoy its results only if you *do the hard work* of getting along with each other' (James 3:18, *The Message,* my italics).

Getting on together, and living and working in real community is not easy. But the payoff and potential are *huge*. It is totally worth it. But we have to recognise that some of the people involved in running those communities carry a significant amount of extra stress.

Too often our response to these sometimes stressful environments is one of three things. We either **walk out**, indignant at what we are expected to put up with; **bail out**, panicked that maybe all that stress is a sign that something is wrong; or **zone out** and carry on in spite of the stress. If things are generally going well for you in your church life, research shows you will happily tolerate high stress for a fairly long time. But this doesn't mean that it has no impact on you physically – or emotionally.

The truth is that what we need to do is **watch out**! We must be aware, and learn how to do the hard work without it taking a big toll on our physical or emotional health. If we want to achieve our potential – and help the groups and people we are working with achieve theirs, we need to be good and handling stress.

Over to you ...

How do you think *you* would define *stress*?

How does stress affect you most?

Where would you place yourself on the following lines?

Not at all prone to   VERY prone to
stress   stress

_____

Not all stressed   Totally stressed out

_____

How do you think your 'church life' affects your stress level? Why/how?

Has stress *limited* you or *stopped* you from doing anything in the last 6 – 12 months?

Is there anything you would you do if you could take stress out of the equation that you haven't been able to do/can't consider doing because of stress?

2

All about *stress*

Now that we have thought about what stress *really* is, let's spend some time thinking about how our stress response system actually works - and how it enables us to respond to the challenges of everyday life. How does stress actually affect us - and when does this become a problem?

In the last chapter we thought briefly about some of the physical and physiological changes that are triggered in our body by the stress response. Now I'm going to simplify those so that we can understand better an important distinction between short-term (acute) stress and long-term (chronic) stress.

Your stress baseline

 Imagine, for a moment, someone standing in a pool of water. At the moment the water level is nice and low - lapping around their ankles. Imagine that the water you (or whichever person you are thinking of) are standing in is around ankle level. Think of that water level as representing the level of stress you are experiencing - both emotional stress and the genuine physical changes it triggers. We all have a stress 'baseline' - the level our stress is at on a normal day.

At this level stress is pretty manageable. Your body is perfectly designed to operate well at this low baseline. Life feels fairly balanced and calm.

Stress 'waves'

Now imagine that something interrupts the peace of your day. You suddenly realise the door is open and the dog has got out, or you remember today is your wedding anniversary and you forgot to get a card, or one of your children comes in and starts yelling at you. This is like a wave in the pool of your stress level as your system responses with a 'spike' of stress.

Again, right now this is fairly manageable. Your baseline is low so you can manage even fairly dramatic waves of stress without too much trouble. And once peace returns, your stress levels quickly fall back to baseline.

Life's 'challenging' phases

 Now imagine that for some reason you are experiencing slightly higher than usual stress for a short but defined period of time. Life throws these sorts of things at us all the time – maybe you have a big project on the go at work, or you're in the middle of a period of exams, or you're planning a big occasion like a wedding. So long as the level of increase in your stress level isn't too high, again this is very manageable. In fact slightly higher levels of those hormones – even the longer term mediators of stress like cortisol – can be useful: we tend to perform better under slightly raised levels than at our baseline. You might be a bit more prone to 'overreacting' to smaller challenges in your day, but overall this raise can actually help you with your studying, planning, moving house, adjusting or whatever it is you are up to.

Then when these little dramas have run their course, things can get back to normal – and once you're back into your everyday routine, your stress levels will return to their baseline.

A Very Bad Day

 Now imagine another scenario. This is a day that started out at your usual baseline, but then went from bad to worse. You realised you forgot that anniversary, then the car broke down, then one of the kids had to come home early from school with a bug, your boss announced he wanted you to present some sales figures to him by the end of the day and your computer decided to crash.

On days like that (we've all had them!), a series of stress 'spikes' happen one after another. Each one raises the water level slightly, and if there is no time between them for you to catch your breath, they can all add up. If life throws too much at you all at once, you can find your stress levels rise quite quickly.

Crisis

Now, time for a quick aside – it doesn't matter who you are and how well you manage stress, we all have what you might call a 'crisis level'. This is where stress levels have risen so high they are right on the verge of exceeding our capacity to cope. Put simply, you are about to lose it. This is when the water level has risen so high that it is now dangerously near your mouth and nose – you might even feel like you are standing on tiptoe trying to keep from going under. When you reach this point you are likely to experience some warning signs. These will be both physical (e.g. heart pounding, headache, breathing fast) and emotional (feeling on the verge of tears, fleeting thoughts of running away, etc.). When you are at crisis level it does not feel very comfortable.

These are the moments in life when it feels, just for a moment, like your nervous breakdown is just round the corner. But they are usually fleeting. In that moment the slightest thing can push you over the edge and you may well find that you do lose it and shout, cry or simply experience an overwhelming need to be where other people are not. But once you do manage to escape somewhere calm, levels will quickly fall back to normal and you will feel much more sane. Hopefully then given a calmer evening, you should be back to baseline and back on an even keel by the next day.

Note that different people find different things trigger their stress waves. This means that some people are much more prone to feeling overloaded or getting very stressed out very quickly.[1]

Raised baseline

Bad days are bad, but they are just short term. What happens if that bad day *doesn't* resolve at the end of the day? What if there is something triggering stress spikes *all the time*, and precious little time to let your levels drop back down. What if your 'challenging phase' carries on and starts to become harder and harder to handle? What if something else starts to happen on top of those things which makes things worse - you start to find it hard to sleep for example (a real classic in quickly making stress problems worse).

What we're describing here is very common, and it is when the actual *baseline* level of stress starts to rise - i.e. even when things are 'calmer', your stress levels do not drop right back down. So, the water level stays higher - say around your knees, or waist, or shoulders ….

The problem with a raised stress baseline is that these things are rarely static. What I mean is that once your baseline goes up it often carries on creeping up, and things get gradually more and more difficult to deal with - just day to day, never mind when those stress waves hit. This is likely to have an impact on

---

1   If this sounds like you, check out Chapter 3 'Are you a stresshead?!'.

you – life is much harder work when you are waist high in stress, and some things become much more difficult – controlling your emotions and sleep are two common examples.

Another problem with a raised baseline is that stress waves can start to become much more problematic – even the smaller challenges of life can trigger a wave, which means that your stress 'water' level starts to get dangerously high. You might feel at risk of being engulfed by your stress, and start to struggle with feelings of panic. When life gets like this people usually feel all too aware of the pressure they are under, but at the same time often feel very powerless to do anything about it. And of course, if things keep on being that stressful, the baseline can itself become alarmingly high. Once your stress 'water' level is up around your neck you start to feel that you are living life 'on the edge'. Here people are very prone to starting to use less than positive strategies to try to help them cope with their stress levels – excessive alcohol for example. It is a very uncomfortable place to live because even a small thing could literally push you under. This is life on the edge of burnout – but it's surprising how many people do live like this, and for how long they are able to keep going.

The impact of chronic stress

So, what if you are living with that chronically raised stress baseline? Some people love to live stress-filled lives and to push themselves that hard. If they feel perfectly happy is there any harm in that?

The problem is that your body simply wasn't designed to live like this. The stress response was designed as a short-term thing to deal with short-term challenges. Chronic stress results in raised levels of those stress hormones – and means that the way your body works is dramatically changed. This has an impact both physically and emotionally.

Let's think about those two main groups of changes triggered by chronic stress:

I. Brain changes

We tend to think of stress as a very emotional thing. It is at the root of the stress system, and the first hormone to be released when it is triggered is actually in the brain. The physical changes that are triggered in the body are triggered by changes first occurring at brain level. Stress doesn't just change how your body operates; it can change the way aspects of your mind operate as well. It causes very real physiological changes in the way the brain operates, and changes how messages are sent between nerve cells and systems in your mind.

Emotional impact

First of all stress has an impact on your emotions, and particularly on the emotions which are controlled by a part of your brain called the amygdala. This is a complex relay system in your brain, the job of which is to identify significant situations and to trigger appropriate emotions in order to make sure you make the appropriate response. The amygdala primarily controls emotions like fear and anger – the ones which are so involved with that fight or flight stress response.

Under chronic stress, the emotional impact is partially dependent on your personality. Some people find that their emotions start to buckle very quickly under chronic stress. The amygdala can become hypersensitive – a bit like putting your brain on red-alert – resulting in an emotional 'fragility', the feeling that emotions like fury or panic are close at hand and could happen at any moment or be triggered by a small thing. In this state it becomes much harder to think rationally about the world around you because your emotions have you constantly on the edge. These tendencies can be particularly hard if you live or work in situations where you usually need to control your emotions well in order to function – parenting or teaching, for example, or in a caring profession.

This increased emotionality means that some people find that under stress they find social situations, or anything that is too 'busy' and stimulating (e.g. busy/crowded rooms, noisy places) very difficult to cope with. They may even trigger intense emotions like panic – along with very strong physical symptoms. This can be a very real problem, particularly if what is triggering your panic is something everyday like going to work, or getting your shopping done. It can also make people prone to hiding away and leave them at risk of becoming isolated. Isolation tends to increase stress levels, taking people away from the things they would usually find helpful – like talking things over with friends. This kind of withdrawal can also be a symptom of depression, particularly if it is accompanied by simply not finding things fun anymore that previously would have been enjoyable. It can very quickly feed levels of anxiety which can become problematic and lead to people being trapped in their own homes.

So, stress is something that puts our emotional selves under intense pressure, and as such it tends to bring out any vulnerabilities that we might have inherent in our personalities.[2] Stress can also directly trigger some problems as people slip into unhelpful strategies to try to help them cope with their emotions, and has been linked to problems like addictions, self-harm and eating disorders, as well as episodes and relapses of conditions like bipolar disorder and schizophrenia.

Memory

Of course the impact of stress on the brain affects much more than just our emotions. Our memory can take a big hit. You know how it feels when you are running round like a mad thing,

---

2   For more about this check out Chapter 3, 'Are you a stresshead?!'

multi-tasking and trying to get at least three hours' of jobs done in one hour? Then you run upstairs to get something ... and can't remember what it was. Or someone tells you their name or phone number and you know - you just *know* - you won't remember it even a few minutes after they told it to you.

In fact, what we might call 'everyday' levels of stress *increase* our memory - luckily for all those students cramming for their exams. But the longer you are stressed, the more it becomes difficult to remember things, not just because your memory is affected but because your attention is all over the place. Negative emotions (which you tend to experience more of in stressful periods) do strange things to your memory too, making it much easier to bring to mind other times when you felt the same emotion. This might be helpful if it reminds you how you escaped the last bear who tried to eat you but it is less useful if you are prone to depression and suddenly find yourself overwhelmed with difficult, sad memories because it can feel like your life is totally overwhelmed by such moments. This little memory 'trick' contributes to the sometimes suffocating hopelessness that can be triggered by depression.

Sleep

Another major cognitive activity that can be disrupted by stress is sleep. The functions of sleep are fairly well debated, but there is a definite consensus that sleep is essential. In fact, attempts for the Guinness Book of World Records to stay awake for long periods of time had to be stopped when the potential dangers of sleep deprivation became better understood – it turns out we can die from lack of sleep.

The real problem with the relationship between sleep and stress is that lack of sleep, or being sleep deprived or unable to sleep for some reason, is actually a strong trigger to your stress system. Sleep is such a basic biological need that overcoming that natural urge is hugely stressful, even if the reason you are not going to sleep is a good one. Therefore people who are operating in situations where they sometimes have to remain awake when they would rather sleep are immediately and inevitably juggling high levels of stress. It doesn't matter whether that is an inherently stressful cause: a newborn baby for example; or something more fun like a party; or mundane, like shift work.

The stress of lack of sleep is particularly unfortunate when you consider that it is much harder to get to sleep when you are under stress. Because stress increases your level of 'arousal' – i.e. how 'awake' your brain is – you will find it much harder to 'switch off' when under stress than normal.

These two links between sleep and stress can very quickly form a vicious circle. Feeling under pressure, busy and tired, you leap into bed and try to go to sleep. But the stress keeps your brain much more active, and it may be very difficult to stop those thoughts buzzing round your brain. Very quickly this can itself lead to triggering emotions like frustration, which make it even harder to go to sleep.

The big issue with sleep is that although it is a very unconscious thing (you can't 'make' yourself go to sleep), it can very quickly become something your conscious interferes with (it is very easy to 'make' yourself unable to get to sleep). About three-quarters of episodes of insomnia have stress as the trigger. The lack of sleep caused by insomnia together with the particular emotional anguish it can trigger often have a very dramatic impact on stress levels. Sleep is a regular 'down time' for both our emotions and our bodies and without it, both can quickly become overwhelmed by the demands placed upon them.

Appetite

We've talked about some of the metabolic changes associated with stress, but of course so much of what you eat and drink is moderated by your mind. Stress increases your appetite – a genuine biological change triggered by all those stress hormones – but what exactly you eat may be more a factor of your emotions than your biology. We tend to eat high sugar, calorie dense 'comfort' foods, – but actually research shows that we don't get any real emotional reward for this type of eating. In fact it often makes us feel worse rather than better. Similarly, the burst of energy given by sugar laden food is short-lived, meaning we can find ourselves hovering near the biscuit drawer again a lot sooner than we intended.

So, some of what we eat is more of an emotional pattern than a biological one, and some studies point to the possibility we can become 'addicted' to certain foods like chocolate. It seems likely that these 'addictions' are emotional and psychological, but this doesn't make them any easier to overcome, and in some cases a real physical effect adds to the emotional strength of our 'need' for these things and makes us even more likely to go for them. Caffeine for example, is a substance that has a significant impact on our bodies and brains, but also is one where very quickly we find that we need more in order to have the same effect. Caffeine 'withdrawal' – when the level of caffeine in your system drops again – can make you feel drowsy, dizzy, and even trigger headaches, meaning that your likelihood of drinking another coffee is much higher.

Other 'vices' show the same mixture of emotional and physical 'cravings'. Drinking and smoking, for example, both have very real physical effects on your body but also are very strong emotional 'coping' strategies, and as such tend to increase in times of stress. You may find that stress triggers other less-than-healthy coping strategies – such as risk taking behaviour, self-harm or disordered eating: things which you feel help you to deal with the emotions you are experiencing, or perhaps make you less likely to have to face those emotions again. Sadly these kinds of strategies often trigger a lot more stress than they ever solve and can go on to become very serious problems.

2. Body changes

At the same time as all those brain changes are going on, chronic stress also has a significant effect on your body. Some people may find that they are not affected that much by stress in terms of their emotions – or that the impact it has on them emotionally simply isn't a big deal. They may even thrive emotionally on the adrenaline charge, and seek out situations where they can live like this. But even those people cannot escape the reality of the physical impact that stress has over time. Note that some physical effects only become apparent after many years – just because you are not aware of them yet doesn't mean they are not happening!

Cardiovascular changes

The main physical changes which can become significant are those that impact the cardiovascular system that moves blood around our body. This system is vital – think of those blood vessels as the motorways of your body, carrying vital cargo to and from your muscles and organs. Under chronic stress, a number of changes affect the way your blood flows. Changes in the tone of the walls of the vessels increase blood pressure, so that blood can be moved faster to where it needs to be. This increased blood pressure can quickly become 'chronic' meaning that it stays high most of the time. Your heart beats more often and harder, and facing this harder work over a long period, the muscle is affected, raising the risk of irregular heartbeats – experienced as 'palpitations' which are even more likely if you drink a lot of caffeine. High blood pressure also increases the risk of a great many serious events including stroke and heart attacks.

Meanwhile metabolic effects – changes in the way you deal with food you have digested – mean that your blood vessels suffer from increased levels of various molecules, mobilised as a quick energy source. These are what you might call the 'wrong kind' of fat. This leaves you at greater risk of your vessels becoming blocked up with these deposits, especially if combined with high blood pressure, which can also damage blood vessels, increasing the risk of blockages and clots forming.

All these effects combined mean that stress is a very real risk factor for heart attacks, strokes and other related problems.

Other metabolic changes

Alongside the mobilisation of fat for energy, another metabolic change is very significant. This is to the chemicals that trigger the release of glucose, and control how fast it can be taken up and stored. Under stress, your body aims to mobilise glucose, meaning that the level of this sugar in your blood will increase significantly. Under normal circumstances if your blood glucose rises too high, your body releases the hormone insulin to reduce it, by stimulating cells to pick up the spare. But under chronic stress, the cells can become less responsive to insulin. This, combined with the spike in blood glucose levels caused by stress can be very difficult for someone with what is called type 1 diabetes - where the body has stopped producing insulin. These people have to calculate how much insulin they need, and inject it regularly. Stress makes this very difficult to control, and often causes problems.

But many cases of diabetes are not related to having enough insulin. In fact it is insulin *resistance* that lies behind a lot of cases of what is called non-insulin-dependent (type 2) diabetes - the kind that people tend to get in their adult years. This is particularly true for those who have put on a lot of weight. All those sugar and chocolate fixes can start to take their toll meaning that your cells have an abundant supply of energy. As a result they simply don't need to take up more glucose and they start to 'ignore' insulin. Over the long term the risk is that this may result in chronically raised blood glucose - type 2 diabetes. This kind of diabetes is a massive problem in our twenty-first-century world. Over 3 million people in the UK are now registered as diabetic, and the majority of these are suffering from this type 2 form of the disease. Diabetes is a serious condition and particularly if poorly controlled, raises the risk of a host of other problems such as cardiovascular disease, kidney damage, or circulation problems so serious it can lead to amputations. In fact 10 per cent of the NHS budget goes on diabetes-related conditions. And a significant proportion of these are related to chronic stress.

Reduced 'housekeeping'

Cardiovascular and metabolic changes are largely down to the increased action of the stress system. But what about its sister system, the one which takes care of all our background 'housekeeping' tasks like digestion? Under chronic stress, this system is significantly impaired, switched off by the constant stress situation. In short, this means a host of things just don't get done as effectively as they should.

Digestion is one clear and immediate victim. Even in your mouth you'll notice the difference as saliva secretion decreases, resulting in a dry mouth and throat. Lower down the impact is mixed – as function in some parts of the bowel is pretty much shut down, while other bits become over-active, with an aim of 'getting rid of' any waste that might be 'hanging around'. All this can result in a chaotic digestive system: stress is linked with symptoms of IBS, and with flare-ups of bowel conditions like Crohn's disease.

Other important systems show decreased activity too – there is good evidence that stress decreases immune function, for example. Catching every bug going? Maybe you need to think about your stress levels.[3]

Stress also has an impact on reproductive systems, generally decreasing your interest in any 'reproductive activity' and decreasing the levels of key hormones like testosterone, which can result in erectile problems for men and delayed or even absent periods for women.

Everyone's different

Of course, what makes the impact of stress so difficult to predict is that everyone is different. What stresses one person out may barely even be noticed by another. What triggers tiny stress waves for me may trigger a stress hurricane for you. But the take home message from the way stress impacts the brain and body is clear: chronic stress is something we need to learn to limit. This kind of stress affects every major system in our bodies, often in significant, dramatic ways.

---

3   An aside on this: Stress can make you more prone to some infections or illnesses, but at the same time we need to avoid slipping into a 'blame culture' whenever people fall ill. If you have been unlucky enough to encounter a nasty dose of flu, a horrible infection or an unpleasant or serious illness the last thing you need is people telling you it is all because you did too much or 'let yourself' get too stressed. Sometimes illnesses just happen through pure bad luck. So let's avoid the temptation to put them all down to stress.

Over to you ...

Imagine YOU were standing in a pool of water – and the water level represents your stress level. Where is the water level NOW? Draw a line on the figure below to show how you are feeling:

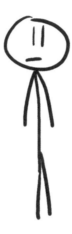

Think about your last week or so. What kind of things can you remember that cause stress 'waves' for you?

Can you recall times when you have come close to *crisis* point?
What did/does that feel like?

Think about the moments when you have some 'down time'
– how low does your water level drop to? Where do you think
your stress baseline is at the moment?

Have you, or has anyone else, noticed any effects of stress on you
– physically or emotionally?

3

Are you a *stresshead*?!

So far we've talked about what stress is – how it is a physiological reality mediated by changes in the levels of your stress system. We've looked at the difference between acute stress, and what happens when your stress system is activated over longer periods of time. Now it's important to take a moment to think about how different people respond to life – and why some of us seem so much more prone to stress problems than others.

What are *your* stress triggers?

It is important to remember that stress is quite an individual thing. Imagine two people go to the same meeting at work. At the meeting it is announced that the company has just won a huge new contract. As the meeting ends, one person leaves ecstatic. The other, however, leaves feeling very stressed. Why? The answer is in their different perspectives – one is going to get the credit for this big new contract whilst the other carries the weight of coordinating and pulling off the response to it and is worrying how on earth s/he is going to do it! We need to realise that our responses to the world around us are mediated by other things going on inside our heads. Your stress responses depend upon the other goals, strategies, beliefs and aspirations that you carry around with you – the very things that make you who you are. Therefore one person's stress nightmare could be another person's great day.

Imagine your head as a bit like a computer. In fact trying to create a computer which acts just like a human brain is a branch of artificial intelligence (AI) research. Now, in order to simplify the complex world in which you exist, your brain needs to take some short cuts. Even those working in AI have found this – unless you put into your computer some kind of algorithm which simplifies all the decisions required moment to moment, the computer is quite simply overwhelmed with all the calculations it needs to make. Think about it – if you decided your every move based on a purely rational analysis of the world it would take a while. Do you fancy toast or cereal this morning? Tea or coffee? These kinds of decisions do not generally need to be made by mathematical calculation and if you did try to view everything in that way, you'd be paralysed in indecision.

In your brain, emotions help you make a lot of these decisions. Contrary to popular belief, they don't act *against* our rational thought processes, but help them out, stopping them from becoming overwhelmed and leaving them to get on with the more important stuff. Whoever you are and whatever your life has been so far, you have acquired a set of goals and rules which you live by, and it is these which influence your emotions and feelings on a day to day basis.

Some of these 'goals to live by' are pretty universal. The goal of aiming to stay alive, for example, is one that most of us carry around day to day. In fact, if your brain detects a situation that might conflict with a goal this serious, it can trigger an almost reflex-like response which has been called emotional hijack.

Hijacked?

Emotional hijack is a key concept, and it will come up a few times in this book, so let's take a moment to think about what it is.

In normal circumstances, your emotions act alongside the part of your brain that likes to think things through rationally. So, do you fancy a piece of cake with your coffee? Emotionally, the response is a big YES, because as a general rule you like cake and it does go well with coffee. Your emotional response biases what your eventual choice will be - but it doesn't have the final say. Part of the emotional response is to trigger your thinking brain to analyse the decision in more depth. So, if you are trying to eat healthily and you already had a couple of biscuits earlier on, you might decide to say no to that piece of cake and over-rule your emotional instinct.

This is a fairly mundane example of those two systems - emotion and thinking - helping you to make a decision, but the same thing happens on a bigger level throughout your life. In contrast to this, emotional hijack is what happens when you need to act *immediately* - when you don't have time to think about what to do. It is a term that was coined in the 1990s by Daniel Goleman.[1] Emotional hijack occurs when your brain uses a strong and immediate emotional reaction to snatch your attention away from whatever else you are doing. At the same time it uses a nerve shortcut to trigger a very quick response - actually *bypassing* your thinking centre. This means it triggers a reaction *before* you have had time to think. About to step out in front of a bus? Emotional hijack means you will jump out of the way before you have even processed what is going on.

This shortcut is generally reserved for critical situations and is accompanied by strong bursts of anger or fear. But it isn't always reliable. Hijack occurs when your brain detects a situation that *may* conflict with a crucial goal. It is the system responsible for what happens when you see something on the floor you *think* is a spider, scream and run away … only to realise at second glance

---

1 Daniel Goleman is a psychologist who in 1995 wrote the very popular book, *Emotional Intelligence*. It is in this book that he first used the term 'emotional hijack'.

that it is the green stalk off the top of a tomato. In this situation the error is unfortunate – embarrassing even if you were spotted, but not crucial. However, emotional hijack can be responsible for more significant unfortunate actions, defined and triggered by key goals you have learned to live by. Found yourself acting on a strong emotion which feels almost like an instinct? Done something you wish you hadn't? Sometimes what we do when we are under the influence of powerful emotions is not what we wish we had done with the benefit of hindsight.

The rules you live by

So what does all this have to do with stress? Stress is strongly associated with the emotions mediated by the amygdala – fear, anger, frustration, etc. The amygdala identifies situations or combinations of things going on around you which might be significant in more serious, significant ways, and if it does identify something potentially important, it uses those emotions and the physical symptoms they are associated with to grab your attention and make sure you focus on the things that matter.

So, when a friend of mine had a hire car and was just filling it up with petrol before dropping it back off, she wasn't really paying much attention until suddenly she realised she felt really anxious. Her stomach was in knots, she felt a bit shaky. Why? She described to me how she 'came to' and wondered what was making her feel that way. Then, when she looked more closely, she realised she was putting unleaded petrol into the diesel hire car. Oops. Sometimes your brain uses emotions as its way to get you to realise something is going on that you need to check out in more detail.

These emotions may or may not be useful, alerting you to helpful things, or less helpful ones, causing you to obsess about something you know that you need to let go or triggering hijack type reactions without letting you think. But either way, the triggers have their physiological impact through that same stress system: the sympathetic nervous system. So, the more prone you are to having emotions like fear and anger triggered, the more stress you are likely to deal with day to day. And how much negative emotion you experience may well come down to the rules you have learned to live your life by, which determine when those emotions are triggered.

Imagine for a moment, a child growing up in a family where things were a bit difficult. Imagine that this child's parent was prone to becoming very angry, unpredictably, possibly even violently at times. We set a lot of our basic 'rules of life' during our childhood. In fact your brain is literally shaped by your experiences, linking things in a very 'cause and effect' way. So this child, trying to learn what triggers these angry outbursts, learns that the best thing to do is to be as invisible as possible. One of the rules they learn to live by becomes that they should never draw attention to themselves. Imagine the same person, now grown up, is asked to lead a discussion in a work meeting. Do you see how those two things clash? The rule - stating they should not draw attention to themselves - and the situation, which requires them to be the focus of the moment are in conflict. This is going to be a very stressful time for them as their brain will trigger anxiety in order to alert them to the clash - much more than it might be for someone who doesn't share the same experiences and the same rules.

Personality - What's your type?

Of course it isn't just your experiences growing up that set the rules that you live by. Some - or at least a tendency to some - are set by your personality. Your personality is the filter you experience the world through, and most psychologists agree that personality varies along certain characteristics - called *traits*. Research has shown that certain personality traits are much more commonly associated with stress than others.

Think, for example, about the most commonly discussed personality trait - extraversion-introversion. This is a fairly well-known trait because it is found on almost all theories of personality. It is also one which is generally accepted to have a biological basis, and is related to what the normal 'baseline' of activation is in your brain. Some people's base activation is fairly high. Their brains 'tick over' at a higher level. This means that they do not need a lot of external 'stimulation' to feel 'alive'. Drama, noise, fuss and bother are generally not pleasant for them and they prefer to seek out quiet, calm spaces where there are not too many people. Given a day on their own they are blissfully happy, not perturbed at all by the lack of interaction. This is a classic introvert. Note that this is nothing to do with confidence, or anxiety. An introvert is not someone who is socially anxious, or awkward. This is just someone who at a biological level does not need a lot of things going on around them in order to be content. And who in fact prefers, on the whole, to live in a calmer space.

Now compare this person to someone who has a base level of activation which is low. This person thrives on energy, drama, adrenaline and excitement. Effortlessly sociable, they are able to chat with several different people at once, moving between conversations and groups without any difficulty. They love the rush of busy-ness, the buzz of big groups of people and the chaos of parties. Given a day on their own they struggle. Their instinct is to seek input and activity. This extravert will experience stress in very different situations to our introvert. In fact the situations which would be calming and soul feeding to the introvert risk being stressful to the extravert! For these two people their personality will have a strong influence on their stress levels - and it could go either way. On the whole though, it is introverts who struggle more, as their work and social lives can push them into spaces which are classically quite stressful for them. They may also find themselves relying on potentially unhealthy or stress-magnifying strategies in order to help them function in more classically 'extravert' environments – things like caffeine, for example. [2]

Another very interesting personality variable in the field of stress is that of perfectionism. This describes something about the level of expectation you have of yourself, the people you love, and the world around you. Someone who scores highly on measures of perfectionism expects those things to be perfect, or near to perfect, all the time. If they are not, they experience stress – emotions like anxiety or frustration are very common.

Perfectionism is a fascinating personality trait. Over half of the population shows some features of it, and in fact it is something that is associated with great potential – most people who are very successful would be categorised as perfectionists, and many famous sportspeople, entrepreneurs and experts in other categories are self-confessed perfectionists. But perfectionism is also strongly associated with less positive things like stress, negative emotions, and emotional and mental ill health. In fact some conditions are so strongly associated with perfectionism that some psychologists have even suggested perfectionism itself should be considered a mental health *problem*. Most, however, are content to think about how perfectionism can be problematic and to talk about what is called 'clinical perfectionism' to describe perfectionism which is having a negative impact on someone.

The problem with perfectionism tends to come from two possible directions. The first is the simple frequency of situations where someone who is a perfectionist will experience stress. Imagine that in order to be happy you have to have a totally

---

2 I find that very often people who come to me seeking help for stress are consuming high levels of caffeine. This magnifies many of the physical impacts of stress and can cause its own physical problems. More and more I am seeing a link between caffeine use and people with a base personality which is quite introverted, but who need to work in more classically 'extravert' environments. They use caffeine not just for energy but to make them more outgoing, expressive and 'out there'. Ask yourself why you need the caffeine – is it just to wake you up or is it something more basic about the way you appear to other people?

and utterly 100 per cent perfect day. Now think about when you last actually *had* one of those days. Perfectionists are often normal humans trying to be super people – trying to achieve just that little bit more than is possible. This means that the more of a perfectionist you are the more stress you will experience, just with getting through your normal day-to-day life. But perfectionists tend to push themselves very hard, so normal day-to-day life is often less than what they expect of themselves, and they often take on way more, pushing themselves relentlessly and keeping on going when others would have stopped long ago, driven by this desire for perfection.

The other problem for perfectionists however is if they slip into the convenience of basing their self-esteem and self-worth on being perfect. Many perfectionists – generally very intelligent and successful people – have never actually failed by real world measures. They tend to excel at whatever they do, and avoid things they are not good at. This means it is all too easy for them to start to think of themselves in terms of what they achieve. All too easily they can become *what they do* instead of *who they are*. And once you start to live by a rule that says 'I am good and acceptable *because I am successful*', you are no longer just desiring perfection – you *need* perfection. Life becomes more stressful because the consequences are much more serious.

Perfectionism can also become something that people use in order to cope with anxiety – and remember that in general as stress levels rise, so do anxiety levels, because at a hormonal level they are so similar. In these situations someone who has a tendency to be a perfectionist can instinctively start to try to 'tick off' things to check that all is perfect – and only then do they allow themselves to relax. The problem here is that those things which need to be perfect before you can relax tend to grow, as can the routines of checking them. Living like this can very quickly become exhausting as you become overwhelmed with the amount of things you have to keep doing to a very high level, and as time to relax becomes more and more rare.

Your personal stress filter

What is interesting about all of these differences in how certain people see the world is the impact that they might have on an individual's stress response. Let's say that we expose a group of people to the exact same stress response – a painful electric shock for example. (This has actually been done and is a good reason why you should always check what you are saying yes to before volunteering to take part in a piece of research!) When we measure the stress response, it turns out that not only do different people have different degrees of stress response, but also that we can influence their stress response by changing their thinking about the trigger. So, if we teach them a technique to cope with the pain, distract them, or even just explain more clearly what is going to happen so it isn't a nasty shock, we can decrease their stress response.

What all this tells us is that the amount of stress you experience isn't just controlled by what life throws at you. It is possible to filter stress through your own thinking. The way you see the world affects the way you experience what it throws at you! This may not sound like good news – because it can explain why some people seem so much more prone to stress than others. But it actually is *very* good news, because it means that if you are struggling with stress, we can help you deal with it better by understanding any thought patterns which may be magnifying your response to life's challenges, and by teaching positive approaches to stress.[3]

So *are* you a stresshead?

Whether they are triggered by personality, by preference or by experience, the thing about the goal structures in your head is that once those basic 'rules to live by' are decided, you tend not

---

3   Much more about that in Part 2 of this book!

to think about them very often – if at all. In fact most of us as adults are unaware of these 'rules' or 'goals' which determine the way we respond to the world around us. But you may well be aware of the level of stress you seem to experience. Some people find that they are much more vulnerable to stress than others. In fact it may be that even what you might think of as 'normal' levels of stress can become problematic to some people. I have lost count of the number of times people have asked me why they seem so affected, when other people seem to be able to manage so much more without being much more than slightly ruffled. The answer may well be in the goals you are living by.

Emotional bonfires

Of course there is another important way in which emotions, and the stress they generate, can start to become problematic. Think of your emotions as a bit like striking a match. When your brain detects something going on that is significant, they flare up, designed to grab our attention, get us to focus on what is going on and make a decision about whether there's anything we need to do or change. Then, once the emotion has done its job, like a match it dwindles and dies out.

The problem for many of us is that this isn't the way we tend to experience emotions. Unfortunately, when your emotions stimulate the parts of your brain that do the analysing and thinking, instead of conducting a nice rational analysis of the situation, they sometimes also trigger a whole cascade of other thoughts, some of which are not very helpful at all. They might include thoughts related to our personality ('I really should be able to get this right every time'), our beliefs or goals ('I'm just useless') or anxieties stemming from our past experiences ('This whole day is just going to be a disaster now'). Instead of helping us deal with the situation in hand, they trigger further emotions.

If that initial emotion was a match, thinking like this is a bit like having a brain full of emotional kindling – balled-up paper, dry twigs and leaves which catch fire very quickly, meaning that one emotional match soon creates a huge blaze – a bonfire. Emotional bonfires are disproportionate in their intensity. They are what happens when someone says something a bit thoughtless and even though we know they didn't mean it, we feel tears pricking at our eyes. They are why one small thing can push us into a negative thought spiral that can ruin our whole day. They last much longer than 'normal' emotions and can smoulder, turning into dark moods which can go on for days or even weeks.

Perhaps most difficult about emotional bonfires is what they do to our experience of, and beliefs about, emotions. They turn emotions from rational, short-term, measured, useful things into dramatic, unpredictable, irrational experiences where we are totally at their mercy. People who experience a lot of these emotions often describe how they feel engulfed by them, they are like waves that hit them, time and time again without warning, and they are powerless to do anything but hunker down and hope that they lift eventually. Bonfire emotions are much harder to understand and trace to their root. They can leave people feeling that they are weak, or vulnerable – that there is something 'wrong' with them. They are hugely stressful. Very often the same people who tell me they are weak and stupid have lived for years under the impact of these difficult, painful emotions. They are the strongest people I know. But eventually even the strongest person buckles under this kind of weight.

Need a brain transplant?

So, what do you do if you suspect that a lot of your stress comes from who you are and how you react? Don't worry – the solution isn't about changing who you are. In fact it is really important that we don't start to think about there being something 'wrong' with who we are. The Bible is very clear that we are created deliberately and personally by God. There are no accidents here:

God 'knits us together' in our mother's womb (Psalm 139:13). This isn't just a physical knitting – it includes your mind and the way you react and respond to the world. All those differences are what make us so fascinating as humans. And they are very key in how we work together in community.

You see, it's easy to take shortcuts when we think about our personalities and the people we are. And it is so much easier to be critical of ourselves than realistic. In part that's because of a real cognitive bias (brain shortcut): we are naturally inclined to focus more on our shortcomings than on the things we do well. After all, those things tend to be more important in terms of trying to avoid making a hash of them again the next time – our brains are biased to try to learn from our mistakes. But in personality terms this can itself be a big mistake! Every personality trait has both a negative side – and a positive one. You might be a bit of a perfectionist, but you will also be excellent at motivating yourself and getting things done. You might be prone to anxiety, but you are also conscientious and reliable. You might be sometimes a bit lazy or struggle to get yourself going, but you work well under pressure where many might find it too much.

We need to understand ourselves wisely before we start to pick holes in who God made us to be. And we need to stop feeling pressure to correspond to some kind of 'ideal personality' when in fact what God created is amazing, wonderful and potential-filled diversity. Paul puts it perfectly in his fantastic advice in Romans 12:5: 'So since we find ourselves fashioned into all these excellently formed and marvellously functioning parts in Christ's body, let's just go ahead and be what we were made to be, without enviously or pridefully comparing ourselves with each other, or trying to be something we aren't' (from *The Message* translation).

We need to stop feeling like we need to change who we are. But how might we need to adjust our thinking? This is Paul's advice in Romans 12: that you 'let God transform you into a new person by changing the way you think' (Romans 12:2

NLT). Studies looking at problematic personality characteristics like perfectionism are very interesting. They tend to look at a group of people suffering with a mental health problem like an eating disorder, and measure perfectionism before and after/ during recovery. What they show is that actually overall levels of perfectionism don't change much. What does change is the way that these tendencies demonstrate themselves – how they influence our thinking. People who 'recover' from unhealthy kinds of perfectionism have learned how to stop it from having a negative effect on them. They have identified, studied and understood what the 'Achilles heel' of their personality might be – their most likely weak point – what, for them, might give way in moments of high stress and pressure and cause them trouble. And then they have learned how to manage it.

In many ways this is the root of what is called cognitive behavioural therapy (CBT), which helps people understand the way in which their thinking, and the goals, rules or beliefs that underlie their thinking patterns, might be triggering problematic emotions, or fanning the initial emotional spark into a huge bonfire. It helps someone understand the difference between the person God made them and the way their own thoughts and beliefs make them feel. In this way, CBT can help you to understand when your being prone to stress is something that you need to learn to manage; e.g. if you are naturally an introvert, but find that the situations you are in a lot of the time are quite stimulating and busy and therefore stressful for you, and when it is something that you need to work on, perhaps by understanding what is feeding emotional bonfires.

So, if you know that you are more prone to stress than some other people, take a moment to examine the way you think. You are not are at the mercy of your own emotions – through becoming more self-aware you can take back control. By starting

to change the way you think, you may well be able to modify
your own stress response.[4]

---

4   Want to learn more? If you are interested in learning more about yourself,
    and the way that your thoughts or goals might be influencing the way
    you experience stress, there is a free course available online. *Life to the Full*
    is a free online course by Chris Williams, an expert in CBT. It takes you
    through, step by step, a course designed to help you think about the way
    your thoughts might be affecting you and triggering stress, anxiety and
    depression. A version of the same course, *Life to the Full - with God*, offers
    some additional thoughts and insights for Christians doing the course. Find
    the course at www.llttf.com or, for the version with Christian content,
    http://www.mindandsoul.info/Groups/196758/Mind_and_Soul/
    Course/Course.aspx).

Over to you ...

Think about the last few times you felt really stressed. Write down briefly what happened/what was going on:

1...

2...

3...

Read the following:

Top ten signs your a perfectionist

1) You can't stop thinking about a mistake you made.
2) You are intensely competitive and can't stand doing worse than others.
3) You either want to do something 'just right' or not at all.
4) You demand perfection from other people.
5) You won't ask for help if asking can be perceived as a flaw or weakness.
6) You will persist at a task long after other people have quit.
7) You are a fault-finder who must correct other people when they are wrong.
8) You are highly aware of other people's demands and expectations.
9) You are very self-conscious about making mistakes in front of other people.
10) You noticed the error in the title of this list.

(From http://news.bbc.co.uk/2/hi/health/3815479.stm)

Do you think you are a perfectionist? Why/why not?

If so, how do you think being a perfectionist affects you?

How does it affect the people around you?

Thinking back to those moments when you last felt really stressed, were any linked to perfectionism?

Can you remember any thoughts that were going through your head at the time these events occurred? These may have been practical (e.g. 'If I don't get there soon I will miss the appointment') or more fleeting (e.g. 'I wish I could run away from all of this'/'Why am I so disorganised?') or something else entirely.

1…

2…

3…

Did you get HIJACKED in any of these moments/incidents? If so, what happened – and did you feel differently when you were calmer?

If not – why not? Did you do something to escape or change things, or did the situation resolve by itself?

Looking at these examples, can you spot any common/repeated themes/issues/thoughts?

Do you think your responses to the situations generally made your stress level *lower* or *higher*?

4

Is your *passion* stressing you out?

So, we've considered whether there could be aspects of the way you think or see the world that leave you prone to higher stress than other people. But might there be something else about who you are that could leave you prone to stress when you least expect it? I know from my experience that the people I work with on stress-related issues generally have one thing in common - they are incredibly passionate people. Could your passion actually be behind some of your stress?

How would you describe passion? It's a tricky one isn't it - to put into words the emotional enthusiasm that most people have for some things. Passion is something that drives us towards certain aims and goals: it leads us to pursue things uncompromisingly. We are called to be passionate people: to love God 'with all our passion' (Matthew 22:37, *The Message*), and promised that that passion will keep us going through tough times. The strength of love that underlies our passion is an incredibly, godly, powerful force. 'The passion of love bursting into flame is more powerful than death, stronger than the grave' reminds the poetic wisdom of the Song of Solomon (Chapter 8:6, CEV). As Christians we want to be passionate for the things that God is passionate about.

We want to be driven, our motivation to be the same as God's. We want to love and care deeply (see Romans 12:10).

So, passion may seem to be universally positive. After all, how can being enthusiastic ever be bad? But our English word 'passion' actually stems from an old Latin verb meaning to suffer. And one look at how Christians describe their passion reveals a focus on something which doesn't necessarily sound like a positive emotional experience. 'May God break my heart so completely that the whole world falls in', prayed Mother Teresa, and a recent chorus has had many of us singing 'break my heart for what breaks yours'. So what is the link between passion and being heartbroken? Is suffering part of being passionate? And does this influence the way we live as Christians? Is passion a positive thing, or can it have elements which are stressful?

Passion and 'godly sorrow'

Passion can come from many different roots. Seeing people's situations and being moved to want to change them for the better can be a very strong motivation and a great reason to be passionate about a cause. This compassion[1] can trigger some very strong negative emotions – grief or sadness for someone's situation for example. The Bible calls this 'godly sorrow' (2 Cor. 7:10, NIV), and notes particularly how it drives passion: 'You're more alive, more concerned, more sensitive, more reverent, more human, more passionate, more responsible' (2 Cor 7:11, *The Message*). Put simply, because you care so much, you are likely to find that this triggers some negative emotions – and this likelihood increases where the situations you are working with are more traumatic, painful or distressing for those directly involved.

---

1 Much more about compassion and empathy in the next chapter, 'Can you care too much?'.

Godly sorrow is driven by the level of compassion we feel for people, i.e. just how much we care, but it also reflects our awareness of things being far from the way God would wish them to be. Paul, in his letter to the Corinthians, explains to them that, 'The thing that has me so upset is that I care about you so much – this is the passion of God burning inside me!' (2 Cor. 11:2, *The Message*). Godly sorrow means we begin to experience something of the emotions God feels about a situation or person. We can see this in action in Luke 19:41 where Jesus looks out over Jerusalem and weeps. The recognition Jesus feels about what is going on in Jerusalem, how far it is from what God desires for that city and where it was going to take them triggers a real grief for the people. Grief is an incredibly powerful emotion, full of sadness for something that is happening or has happened, but also acknowledging a kind of helplessness as something happens that we desperately wish was not happening. It fuels a furious passion, a desire to stop the same kind of thing being repeated: a desire to change things for the better.

As Christians, the closer we get to God and the more time we spend with God, the more we begin to understand the grief that God holds for how far the world has moved from the way God created it – and the impact that has had on God's people. Of course the grief God holds is way beyond anything we could comprehend or experience. But as we grow in faith we do begin to learn *something* of it. That's where the concept of our heart being 'broken' by an awareness of sin – sometimes our own, but often by witnessing the terrible impact of sin on our world and people – comes from.

So, whatever it is you are passionate about, you may find yourself also experiencing these kinds of emotions: sorrow, pain, grief. Whether or not you find the emotions you experience *emotionally* stressful, it's important to recognise that these are *physiologically* stressful because they trigger a very real physical stress response. It is for this reason that people working in environments where they support people in very difficult or traumatic situations need to be particularly careful about how they handle the inevitable stress of their role. It isn't because they don't like what they do; quite the opposite. Their passion puts them at risk of heightened stress. Emotional pain triggers the same parts of the brain as physical pain: it is physiologically stressful. Therefore we must treat it with respect; we are not designed to operate with that kind of emotion all the time.

Passion and guilt

Godly sorrow is one example of a negative emotion flowing out of our passion. But guilt – another very powerful emotion sometimes associated with passion – tends to operate in a different way: as the *source* of our passion. In contrast to the times when we are passionate about things because of how much we care about them, if we are honest, sometimes our passion for something stems from a desire to be rid of guilt.

Of all the emotions, guilt is probably the most complex. This tricky little emotion can plague us, and it is hard to pin down. How do we define guilt? What is its purpose? Is it a wholly negative thing or can it ever be positive? Guilt is generally defined as the emotion we experience when we feel (rightly or wrongly) that we have done something wrong – by our own inner moral code or by someone else's rules. Its function, thinking about our model of emotions, is to draw our attention to things we have done wrong – things that clash with the rules we aim to live by. It is closely related to shame – in fact some psychologists use the terms interchangeably – except that shame is generally a more public emotion – what we feel if our mistakes or bad decisions become common knowledge – whereas guilt is more of a private, inward emotion.

It is interesting that guilt and shame first appear in the Bible directly after Eve takes her first bite of the forbidden apple, and sin enters the world. Before this we are told that God looks on his creation and sees that it is 'good'. This word, the Hebrew word *tov* means that something is good and beautiful but more than that, it means it is *just as it should be*. God's original creation was just as it should be. It was God's ideal for us. Then something happened. Eve took fruit from the tree 'of the knowledge of good and evil' (Genesis 2:9 - 17, NIV). Intriguingly the name of this tree again uses the same word *tov*, but contrasts it in a very 'black versus white' way with an opposite, evil. Thus creation pre-Eve's actions was all about God's ideal, but afterwards something else was introduced which was far from the way things 'should' be – in fact it was the opposite of what God wanted.

Guilt and shame therefore stem from our awareness of something being 'wrong' compared to God's plan or desire for us. It may relate to a specific law or commandment, or it may be a sense of our own actions having conflicted with what God would want us to do. Guilt is not something that was part of God's ideal – it wasn't necessary then because the things far from his plan simply didn't exist. Guilt isn't sinful; instead it is a necessary product of sin being in the world. It is, one could say, an awareness of things being the opposite of what God would want them to be.

So, guilt is a complex emotion. Sometimes we feel guilt because we are painfully aware of how far we ourselves are from God's ideal. At other times guilt is triggered by something far outside of us – something in the world which is the opposite of what God would want. When we carry this kind of guilt we carry a burden that isn't our own.

The Bible teaches that 'all of creation is groaning' as it 'waits in eager expectation' (Romans 8:19, 22, NIV). More than that, the same passage tells us that 'the creation was subjected to frustration … by the will of the one who created it in hope that the creation itself will be liberated from its bondage to decay and brought into the freedom and glory of the children of God' (Romans 8:20-21). That word in verse 20, variously translated as 'frustration' (NIV), 'vanity' (KJV), 'futility' (NASB), is the same one as used in Ecclesiastes 1 when Solomon cries out 'everything is meaningless' (Ecc 1:1, NIV). It carries that same essence of things being so far from the way God intended them to be! And the key message from Romans 8:19-22 is that our experience of that feeling is designed to push us one way only: towards God and a greater understanding of what God desires for us: freedom from such things and a return to God's ideal. Therefore guilt, when it works, pushes us towards good things, and in that sense it can fuel a very healthy form of passion to see change and an energy moving back towards God's way.

However, like many things in God's creation, in our sinful world guilt can become twisted to have a wholly negative effect on us. If guilt, instead of driving us out of ourselves and towards what God desires, becomes turned inward, it eats us up as we become more and more aware of our own inadequacies. This kind of guilt undermines our sense of who we are. It challenges our intrinsic value and can leave us incredibly vulnerable, as we take the blame upon ourselves. This kind of guilt pushes us into isolation as we withdraw - not just from other people but also from God.

Paul talks about these two very different kinds of distress that guilt can produce in 2 Corinthians 7:10: 'Distress that drives us to God … turns us around. It gets us back in the way of salvation. We never regret that kind of pain. But those who let distress drive them away from God are full of regrets' (*The Message*).

Some people - in particular often those who have experienced great trauma, abuse or suffering often at the hands of other people - carry this kind of guilt even though what they experienced was through no fault of their own. They become convinced that they are the opposite of what God intended - I've heard many people talk of a fear that they are intrinsically 'evil' or 'bad' people. At a lower level, many of us find that our actions, if we are honest, are motivated by guilt rather than compassion. We do what we do, not because we want to but because we need to in order to try to drive away our guilt.

So guilt can drive a form of passion but it is a form that is much less positive. Passion driven by guilt is unrelenting, exhausting, all consuming. It stems from fear and vulnerability and a desperate attempt to drive things away. It can very easily exhaust us because it eats us up from the inside out. It is physiologically and emotionally very stressful. We have to be particularly careful here because from the outside this passion can look just the same as our more positive passion. But it hides a dark secret and is far from healthy.

Passion and frustration

As a psychologist, there's one final emotion I know often goes hand in hand with passion: frustration. Things we feel passionate about trigger strong emotions in us, and the more we care the more we are likely to become irritated when things are not (according to our perspective) done well. In fact, that sense of frustration and irritation with the way things are - research often refers to it as a 'dissatisfaction with the status quo' - goes so hand in hand with passion that it can be a useful clue about something God has made us passionate about and what God may be calling us to.

Levels of passion can also be indicative of our personalities - specifically how emotional we tend to be. People differ in their experience of emotions - how often and how strongly they experience them. It is a common sense link therefore that someone who tends to experience the world in a more emotional way is more likely to be powerfully passionate about something - but the same person is going to be more prone to facing feelings of frustration or despondency when things are not going well.

So what does this tell us about our Christian lives? If we call out to God to make us passionate, we should understand that this means we are also likely to be frustrated. This isn't a bad thing. In fact we are in great company. Jesus experienced and expressed a whole range of emotions during his years of ministry including frustration. More than once he seems to cry out in frustration, usually when people misunderstood or misinterpreted God. 'How long shall I put up with you?' he cried out to his own disciples when they brought him someone they had 'failed' to heal (Matthew 17:17, NIV). 'You brood of vipers,' he said to the Pharisees, 'how can you who are evil say anything good?' (Matthew 12:34, NIV). Experiencing frustration is not a sin, but we must be careful what it leads us to do. 'In your anger do not sin' is sound advice (Ephesians 4:26, NIV). The more passionate we are, the more we need to learn good positive strategies for dealing with frustration.

Be wise

What can we learn then from this deeper understanding of passion? We need to approach our passion with real wisdom.

First, we must be aware of the intensity of our passion and the drive that it can produce. We must make good decisions and set sensible limits according to our very human needs and in spite of our passion. Jesus, as God, was full of passion, but sometimes turned away from the needs of others when he needed to attend to his own needs, or those of his disciples – in order to rest/sleep (e.g. Mark 4:38), eat (Mark 6:31), and pray/connect with God (Luke 5:16). Whether it is frustration or sorrow we need to be aware that we are carrying it, and aware of our need for regular time out.

This is particularly key in light of the negative emotions that passion can trigger, and becomes even more important for those of us working with people or situations that are very distressing/ traumatic. I remember a time when I was working one to one with an expert as part of a course of treatment for a back problem. I was amazed at the accuracy with which she could identify weeks when I had been meeting with people who were acutely distressed or suicidal. The change in the physical tension in my muscles was so strong that she picked up on it immediately. We must never underestimate the impact this stuff can have on us, and we must always be meticulous in the way we make time to relax, debrief or remind ourselves of Gods bigger perspective.

Secondly, we must be self-aware and honest about the roots of our passion. We need to know that passion can sometimes stem from something that actually we need to work through. The need it is meeting is one of our own, rather than the need of anyone or anything else. We need to really carefully examine these things, because the risk is then that our 'passion' can drive us so hard that we exhaust ourselves. If we carry guilt for someone or something else, we cannot fix it by our own actions, no matter how hard we try. That way only leads us to exhaustion. Instead we need to let go of what we carry, because it is not our own.

Don't go it alone

Finally, we need to make sure that we are never trying to be ministry 'lone rangers'. Jesus was God and yet he didn't try to do his ministry on his own. He never sent disciples out on their own either. We need to be aware of the chance that our emotional load might lead to a tendency to isolate from others, and might make it harder for us to connect with God, and we must actively plan times and opportunities to connect. Two things Jesus prioritised during his ministry were time alone to pray and be with God and time with his disciples. We must treat our emotional load with respect and make sure that we look after ourselves as well as looking after the people we care for. Otherwise all too soon we can become in need of care ourselves.

Over to you ...

What would you say are the three things you are *most* passionate about?

Ask your partner/best friend/someone who knows you well what they think you are most passionate about ... did they give the same responses?

Do you identify with the concept of 'godly sorrow'? Is it something you have ever experienced in relation to the things you are passionate about?

Have a think about the things you most often feel guilty about. Note them down below - and ask yourself in each case - is this something in *you* that you feel is far from God's ideal, or something in the *world* that doesn't reach God's ideal?

Then consider - how much is fixing this *your* responsibility? Give it a score from 0% (not your responsibility at all - responsibility is someone else's/God's) to 100% (totally your responsibility).

Do you think you ever carry guilt for things which are not your responsibility/fault? How does this affect your stress levels?

Where would you place yourself on the following line:

I never/rarely get   I get frustrated
frustrated   A LOT

———————————————————————————————

Thinking about what things frustrate you the most, are they linked to the things you are most passionate about?

Are there any things you need to add to the list of what you are passionate about now?

5

Can you *care* too *much*?

Following on from thinking about how the things we are passionate about might contribute to our stress load, there's one final area we need to think about which is hugely relevant for a church context. It is an area which is also central to who we grow to be as Christians, and the way we seek to live with one another. It is about how we care. How might the way you care influence how stressed you are?

It goes without saying that we do want to care. 'Be good friends who love deeply' advises Paul in Romans 12. Jesus himself said that the second most important commandment – after loving God – was to love your neighbour as yourself (Mark 12:29-33). God, after all is 'the Father of compassion and the God of all comfort' (2 Cor. 1:3, NIV). But is it possible to love too much? Can our desire to care for others sometimes have an unexpected impact on ourselves? And might there be healthy and less than healthy ways of caring?

Love without limits?

As Christians it is tempting to want to love without limits – to give ourselves entirely to other people and focus on their needs rather than our own. Gandhi once said that the best way to find yourself was to 'lose yourself in the service of others'. In Jesus we see a model of a human loving and giving perfectly – but importantly we also see limits to that giving. As we've already noted, Jesus sometimes moved away from people in need to pray (see Luke 5:16), to sleep (Matthew 8:24) or to find space for his own emotions (Matthew 14:10–13). So where does the balance lie in how *we* care for people?

One often-used word in this area is that of empathy. Empathy is about more than just understanding what someone is feeling – it involves feeling someone's pain, and communicating to them that you really understand what they are going through. Empathy seems to be a vital skill in human relationships. The element of being able to understand the world from someone else's perspective is a crucial part of social interaction. Understanding why people act and react the way they do is what makes us able to share our space and our lives with them.

Research suggests there is a natural variance in how intrinsically empathetic people are, and such variation may explain why some are more naturally drawn to caring roles or situations. Empathy has been demonstrated to be a really important construct in caring professions like medicine, counselling, etc., but there is a problem. Too much empathy seems to lead to an increased risk of stress, burnout and compassion fatigue.

The roots of why this is the case seem to lie in what empathy involves at a brain level. Empathy is an instinctive ability to place yourself in someone else's position and understand what they are feeling. More than that though, empathy involves an element of mirroring those feelings in what you experience yourself – it involves an emotional reaction *yourself* as you reach out to others. So you don't just understand their pain, to a degree, you feel it as well.

Research investigating this perhaps surprising aspect of empathy has implicated what are called *mirror neurons*. Mirror neurons are an absolutely fascinating discovery in the way our brains work, discovered in the 1990s when scientists realised that there were groups of cells in the brains of monkeys which reacted not just when they did something - grabbing a banana say - but also when they watched another monkey doing the same thing. Experiments soon confirmed that human brains had neurons which acted in the same way. If you watch someone doing something, or even if you imagine performing an action yourself, these cells fire off exactly as though you were actually doing the same thing in real life.

The discovery of mirror neurons triggered a flare of excitement in the scientific world, and theories, debates and suggestions about their role in various syndromes and circumstances still rages. But the role they may play in empathy is very interesting. It turns out that mirror neurons are triggered when we see another human experiencing an emotion, and go on to trigger some kind of experience of the same emotion in us. Although there's still debate amongst experts, this role of mirror neurons suggests that as part of empathy we experience something of what we would literally feel were we in the other person's shoes. We know however that it is their experience, not ours, so that's what makes it empathy.

Emotional burnout?

Bearing this in mind, it's easy to see why too much empathy can be exhausting. If you constantly not just observe, but to some degree *experience* the emotions of others, then you may well be more drawn to try to help them. What we mustn't overlook is that you will also suffer emotional stress from the experience of sharing their pain. For most people this is likely to be minor and manageable - even something they don't notice. There will be a group of people however who are *highly* empathetic, perhaps irresistibly drawn to help others in difficulty - who might talk of how they cannot bear to leave people when they are experiencing pain or suffering, who might be acutely aware of the emotional pain they feel at witnessing the suffering of others. Should these people 'give in' to this urge and spend ever increasing amounts of time in caring roles; should they fail to learn how to limit or sensibly modify their instinctive responses, they will be at risk because of the sheer physiological weight of the emotional stress they themselves will experience as part of their caring.

There is good scientific evidence for this suggestion. Studies looking at empathy within the caring professions clearly link heightened empathy with an increased risk of stress and burnout. Combine that with the fact that heightened empathy responses are likely in those who already demonstrate a tendency to be more emotional themselves and you can see why a very empathetic person working in a caring field could be at risk of issues linked to stress and negative emotion.

Who are you caring for?

Another element that may well be relevant in empathy is that of other individual differences which might make some people much more drawn to be empathetic than others. We've already looked at the way in which our own experiences and personality might influence the way we act and react to the world around us. This applies just as much when you consider how caring we are. In fact many factors determine how caring we are as people – and within that very category there is more variance in terms of *why we care*. It seems that a subset of people, who carry a significant emotional load in the way they care for others, might be at particular risk of a kind of empathetic burnout.

It's always good to ask ourselves why we are doing what we are doing. Caring for others always presents itself as something we do for *them*. But if we're honest sometimes it is really as much about us. We might care for someone in order to stop ourselves feeling guilty. We might care for them in order to stop them being a problem to us or someone else. We might care for them in order to meet one of our own needs – perhaps a need to be needed, or a need to feel good about ourselves. The more intrinsic the need we are trying to meet by caring for others is – particularly if it is one of our own basic needs – the greater the risk that we might go too far in our caring.

Healthy caring

So how should research and understanding like this change the way we care as Christians? What can we learn from the way Jesus lived about how best to love the people around us? What is very interesting is that the Bible doesn't actually talk about empathy. Instead it uses another word which has recently begun to generate a great deal of interest in the research world: compassion.

Compassion is defined in similar terms to empathy as the ability to appreciate the emotions of another. It's not a shallow response by any means – the biblical word translated as compassion literally means to be moved 'from your gut'. There's a clear implication that compassion still involves a real emotional response from us. However rather than just generating that emotional response (as in empathy), compassion triggers a *caring* response – behavioural actions and reactions rather than emotional ones. Compassion triggers motivation and action to relieve or alleviate the suffering that has been observed but also offers a protection from the potentially difficult emotional impact of the suffering of others. This means that someone is able to continue caring for others in a way that is effective and valuable to those in need, but also protects them better from potentially negative impacts on their own wellbeing.

The link between compassion and actions to relieve suffering is clear in the Bible. Matthew 14:14 describes Jesus coming upon a crowd of people in need: 'When Jesus landed and saw a large crowd, he had compassion on them and healed their sick' (Matthew 14:14, NIV). Jesus' compassion is directly and intrinsically linked with his action – he didn't just feel empathy for them, he was moved to act. The Old Testament too shows people moved to act outside the usual reactions of their time because of compassion. In Exodus 2:6, Pharaoh's daughter, in the midst of a time when the Pharaoh himself had ordered all Jewish baby boys to be killed after they were born, found a basket in the river containing just one of those boys. The Bible tells us she 'opened it, and saw the child – a boy, crying! – and *she felt compassion for him* and said, "This is one of the Hebrews' children."' (Exodus 2:6, NET, italics mine). This compassion is what leads her, in the next verse, to ask the child's mother to nurse him and take care of him for her. Compassion does more than stir our emotions – it changes the way we act.

Compassion is also something that is described as a basic component of the character of God – that character which we reflect. God is 'compassionate and gracious' (Psalm 103:8, NIV); and 'full of compassion' (Psalm 116:5, NIV), and it is among the ways that God describes Himself (Exodus 22:27). It's important to note that God's compassion is more than 'just' a feeling. It is God's compassion that moves God to act – whether that be to hear the cries of God's people (as in the Exodus verse), or to show mercy (e.g. Deuteronomy 13:17). We learn that it was because of God's 'great compassion' that God did not abandon the Israelites in the wilderness, in spite of their repeated decisions to turn from God (Nehemiah 9:19, NIV) and that it is compassion which enables God to hold back anger when people sin – meaning it is intrinsically linked with the concept of grace (e.g. Exodus 34:6, Psalm 103:8, 86:15). We too are called to be compassionate in turn (Ephesians 4:32; Philippians 2:1-2; Col. 3:12) – and this will not just be an emotional response but will require motivation and real action.

It looks like our understanding of caring from a clinical or academic approach is starting to catch up with this guidance from the Bible. Recent projects, seeking to value compassion over other forms of caring like empathy, have begun what is termed 'compassion training', seeking to increase skills which trigger a compassionate rather than empathetic response to the suffering of others. Helen Weng, an expert from the Centre for investigating Minds, University of Wisconsin, Madison, described on BBC Radio 4's *All in the Mind* programme back in June 2013, her research into how to train people to become more compassionate.[1] Her meditation-based training asks people to visualise feelings of compassion, and of wishing that their suffering was relieved, first for someone they love in a difficult situation, then for themselves (feeling and allowing ourselves to be compassionate for ourselves is a surprisingly difficult skill) and finally for someone that they do not get on with (it is much harder to feel compassion for someone we dislike).

What is particularly interesting about projects like this looking at the contrast between compassion and empathy is what has been demonstrated to be going on at a brain level. Whilst both activate parts of the brain accosted with processing and understanding the emotions of others, empathy also primarily activates areas of the brain involved in the *personal experience* of negative emotion. Compassion in contrast triggers activation in the areas of the brain focusing on *care or nurturing behaviours*. More than that, in individuals who undergo training in compassion skills, the corresponding empathetic emotional activation of their brains seems to decrease as their compassionate activation increases. Finding action in our response seems to provide a release for some of the elements of our emotional response – that element of an emotion which drives us to act is then channeled into something positive, altering in a key way the impact the experience has on us. These responses demonstrate what could be seen as a more long-term manageable response to other people's pain and trauma. Compassion allows us to appreciate someone else's pain, and support them, without becoming too distressed ourselves. There's also evidence that

---

1 You can listen to this programme at www.bbc.co.uk/programmes/b0213yzy

practicing compassion can have other positive impacts for people
– reducing stress and increasing levels of happiness.

Actions speak louder ...

One thing that is particularly interesting about research into
compassion training is the way in which, when caring, it is not
just our emotional response which is important: actions matter.
It is not enough just to be moved emotionally by someone's
circumstances. We must be moved to act as well. 'Dear children,
let's not merely say that we love each other; let us *show the truth
by our actions*' says 1 John 3:18 (NLT, italics mine). Similarly, James
2:17 says, rather starkly: 'faith by itself, if it is not accompanied
by action, is dead' (NIV). It seems from this recent research
that caring focused entirely on empathy may also have a very
negative impact on us as carers.

Of course we must be careful too of how we act and
what the consequences of our actions are. One of the central
'commandments' of caring is that we must be very careful that
we do not care for people in such a way that supports them
to remain in places which are very unhealthy. Caring should
never encourage people into dependence or allow them to
lose their own sense of being in control of their own future.
Instead our caring should involve actions which empower them
and enable them to move forwards towards better times and
better situations. It is these kinds of action which form part of a
compassionate response.

Caring needs to be about more than instinct

All of these findings from so many different fields therefore must
be allowed to influence what we learn about how to care within
the church. It is so tempting in this area to see something like
caring as just about instinct. We look for those who are natural
'carers' – who seem to automatically seek out those in need,

or who are automatically sought out by the same people. We tend to treat caring as something we either 'have' or 'don't have' rather than as something we need to learn. We need to realise that to care well requires great wisdom and experience as well as good instincts.

For ourselves, caring for others requires us to be very self-aware. The question of why we do what we do is a very important one, particularly for those who are in caring professions. It's something that most good professional training courses cover as a matter of great significance whilst someone is learning to be good at what they do. It is important that we do the same, particularly with those who take up caring roles within our churches. The 'best' carers may not be the ones who care the most!

But most of all, findings like these from clinical research add to the great advice in the Bible to teach some important truths about how best to care for people. It's really important as Christians that we realise that what we're called to isn't an emotionally exhausting, draining, distressing experience. Good caring needn't carry an overwhelming emotional impact for us and our families. We need to recognise that sometimes the people who do experience caring like this – who may often be seen as the 'ideal' of how to be truly caring – may actually need some help and guidance in how they do care for others. We must not promote a form of caring for others that destroys ourselves.

What we're called to as caring Christians is something much more than empathy – something real, but that leads us to desire change – justice, improvements and the alleviation of the suffering of others. If we move from a purely emotional empathetic position to one of action and compassion, we can allow ourselves and the person/people we are supporting to move forwards.

Over to you ...

How would *you* define *empathy* and *compassion*? What do you think is the difference between the two?

Would you describe yourself as a naturally empathetic person and/or compassionate person?

Have you ever experienced a situation where you have felt an emotional pain linked to the suffering of another person? Are there particular situations/circumstances where you experience this?

Particularly if you are in a caring role, do you think (be honest!) that your caring for others meets any needs in you? If so, what are they?

Would you say that your caring is guided by instinct, or by something else? How much do you plan how you respond to the needs of others?

6

Are you *burned out?*

In this first section of the book, we've taken a long hard look at stress and what exactly it is. We've thought about some of the causes of stress, and asked some hard questions about what might be stressing us out. We've thought about signs and symptoms of stress, as well as looking at what some of the short and long term impact of stress might be on us.

Before we move on to look at some practical thoughts on how to manage stress better, it's important that we touch on one last subject. The impact of stress, whether it is physical or emotional, can develop gradually over years. But sometimes stress can build up to such a degree that it stops us in our tracks and forces us to take stock of what is going on in our lives. When this happens, we talk about burnout.

What is burnout?

Burnout happens when our stress levels have become so high that we cease to be able to function in the way we would normally want or hope to. This may be due to physical causes, or emotional difficulties, but often it is a combination of both – and of other factors which barge in and interfere in our lives at a time when we least want them to. Burnout is when our attempts to live as super people are rudely and abruptly interrupted by our very human frailties.

Definitions of burnout vary. It occurs when our capacity to continue working and existing under high stress situations simply runs out. It is about physical and/or emotional exhaustion. Because we are all different, your experience of burnout – or the early warning signs of it if you do not hit full burnout – may well be very different from other people you are close to, but here are some common symptoms which may indicate that you are approaching a point where burnout is a very real risk:

Physical:

- Feeling exhausted: lack of energy, tired all the time
- Frequent headaches, stomach aches, etc.
- Frequent, long duration or just plain 'hard to shift' minor illnesses – colds, infections, etc.
- Worsening of long term conditions such as eczema, irritable bowel syndrome, migraines, etc.
- Palpitations or noticing your heart racing
- Sleep problems: finding it hard to drop off, sleeping very lightly; waking frequently/too early
- Problems with digestion.

Emotional/cognitive:

- Struggling to motivate yourself to do anything
- Lack of enjoyment of things you usually love to do
- Frequent, strong or unexpected bursts of emotions like anxiety, frustration, etc.
- Panic attacks
- Finding it hard to 'switch off' your brain, obsessional thinking
- Tearfulness (often without much of a trigger)

- 'Escape' thinking – suddenly wanting to run away or dreaming of leaving job/home
- Feeling ineffective in everything you do/performing worse than usual at work, etc.
- Struggling to concentrate on anything
- Emotional problems: persistent low mood/depression, anxiety or bursts of anger/irritation
- Memory problems
- Increased reliance on things like alcohol, smoking, etc. to try to relax.

As well as these symptoms you may notice other things about the way you are functioning in your day to day life. Often people find that although it is hard to put a finger on specific things, they simply aren't coping as well as usual. Another well-recognised impact of burnout is on your levels of empathy and caring. Particularly if you work in a caring role – or if your responsibilities at home involve caring for children or elderly relatives – you may find yourself struggling to care about some things, and instead find yourself experiencing feelings like frustration or irritation at situations or needs which you would usually be able to handle.

Too much of a good thing?

The root of burnout is simple: doing too much for too long. Like a car running on fuel, if you burn up too much fuel (emotionally or physically) and don't take enough time to recover those energy reserves, you will eventually run out. However, there are some interesting physiological and cognitive things going on which may well underlie some of your burnout symptoms.

One area which has stimulated a lot of debate surrounds the impact on your body of chronic changes to your usual level of adrenaline. Adrenaline, as you may remember, is usually a short-term hormone secreted as part of your acute stress response. It is a very 'emotional' hormone, mediating much of your response to emotions like anxiety and anger. Adrenaline can also be involved in other physiological responses – for example to illness or infection. A host of theories have sprung up over the years about what happens if we experience sustained high levels of adrenaline. It isn't a hormone which becomes chronically raised in the same way that cortisol does, but if you have too many triggers, those little bursts of adrenaline can all merge together to produce nearly the same effect. Adrenaline release can also be increased in response to certain chemicals – like caffeine for example – so it may be that our own actions when under stress make this effect even more exaggerated.

One theory surrounding burnout is that experiencing too much adrenaline over a long period of time can cause problems. Some theories focus on the impact of long-term high levels of adrenaline – linking a variety of physical and emotional symptoms to this. Others talk about so called adrenal burnout – when your adrenal glands become unable to continue to respond to even small 'stresses', leaving you exhausted and unable to function normally – or look at the impact of a sudden drop in adrenaline once a period of acutely heightened stress lessens off. Such approaches and theories have not yet been proven, and remain controversial, although some approaches to treat burnout, as well as other conditions like chronic fatigue, have grown out of them.

Amid the various debates, what is important to note is that the symptoms we experience when we are burned out are very real, and have their roots in genuine physiological changes in our body and brain They are not 'all in the mind', nor are they about weakness, hypochondria or some kind of 'giving in.' This is very important in terms of how we respond to burnout – our own or that experienced by someone else. Much as we might be tempted to employ a 'get a grip' approach, ignore what is going on and push through it, burnout represents very real exhaustion. You cannot push through it. If you do not take time out to rest and recuperate it is very likely that either your body or brain will force you to do so.

Biblical burnout

One very interesting thing about burnout is just the clear biblical examples of it. After all, the Bible is full of accounts of real people dealing with extreme and dramatic situations. We would expect some of them to struggle with the level of stress they have to manage - and they do! John the Baptist, for example, who was known for his confidence, his single-minded faith and wholehearted approach to his life and ministry. This is the man who strode out of the desert and proclaimed to everyone that the Messiah was coming. The same man who recognised Jesus straight away and baptised him. The man Jesus was talking about when he said 'no one ever born on this earth is greater' (Matthew 11:11, CEV). And yet we hear from this man a bit later, under immeasurable stress and facing his inevitable death in prison, suddenly sounding very different. Luke 7 tells us that as he heard of the spread of news that Jesus was some kind of great prophet, and was performing miracles: healing people and raising the dead, he sent some of his disciples 'to the Lord to ask, "Are you the one who is to come, or should we expect someone else?"' (Luke 7:19, NIV). What's this? John the Baptist suddenly hit by doubt? How can the same man who did all he has done ask this question? This is what stress can do to you, sapping you of your conviction, your confidence, your energy. Jesus responds not with any 'get a grip' philosophy, lecture, trite words or super spiritual talks, but by healing a bunch of people, then telling John's disciples to go back and report that 'The blind receive sight, the lame walk, those who have leprosy are cleansed, the deaf hear, the dead are raised, and the good news is proclaimed to the poor' (Luke 7:22, NIV). Jesus understands John's vulnerability at that time and sends evidence to confirm *what John really knows already*. John's experience of stress demonstrates just how burnout can make you question things that you know to be true – and that this can happen to any of us.[1]

Another perspective the Bible can give us on burnout is whether this is in some way 'desirable' or something we should be aiming for in ministry. I have already explained my frustration at the number of times I have heard people proclaim that they want to 'burn out' for God. There is no biblical precedent for this. In fact the Bible is full of evidence that this is something we should avoid. Consider Jesus, for example. Here we have God on earth for a short, finite period of time. A lot of this time was spent waiting for the time when his ministry was to start. Then there follow a few frantic years before he is put to death on the cross. Given that Jesus knew how it would end we might expect him to have a 'push it to the limit' attitude during those years of ministry – a kind of 'I'm only here for a short time let's chuck out the limits and pack as much in as is possible' approach. But what we see time and time again is Jesus taking sensible steps – for him and for his disciples. Admittedly he pushed the limits, grabbing sleep where he could (on boats for example), and things didn't always go according to plan – people often followed him when he tried to find some time to rest. But what we see is a wisdom-filled, measured approach to his ministry together with an awareness and acceptance of the limitations that being human resulted in. Jesus did not burn himself out – and perhaps we can learn as much from that as we can from the examples of characters who did.

Emotional burnout

Burnout, if it has its impact physically, may be easier to recognise than it is to deal with (more about that later). The impact of illness or physical ill health tends to force us into rest, and much

---

1   We'll look at another great example of biblical burnout, from the life of Elijah, in the second part of the book.

as we may hate it, we have to recognise our own need to slow down. Perhaps more subtle, and certainly more dangerous is the impact that burnout can have on our thinking and emotions.

In thinking about the way your mind works, it is important to recognise the difference between two different kinds of 'fact'. The first is an empirical fact. This is a kind of information that is measurable, quantifiable and reliable, i.e. if someone else measured it they would get the same result. So, the desk I am working on right now is 1 metre 60cm wide. It just is. Whoever measures it, provided their tools and method are accurate, it will still measure the same. The second kind of 'fact' is very different. These are opinions or perspectives on something. So I can say that my desk is 'nice'. You may or may not agree, if you were here to look at it. Now, although these two examples are fairly easy to recognise, some are more tricky. So if I say my desk is 'blue', which kind of fact is this? This could be a fact, were it to be based on some kind of scientific study of the nature of the material my desk is made of – but much more likely is that it is a statement of how I see my desk – so a kind of opinion. It comes from my perspective. Someone else (my husband for example) might think it was green. I could say they were wrong – but in reality we just both have different opinions.

Now consider your own thoughts and emotions. A lot of emotional difficulties come from treating the kind of information they give us as the first kind of fact when in fact what they are is the second. So, if I say that I feel guilty about something, that is my brain alerting me to the *possibility* that I might be guilty – not the absolute fact. If I treat my feelings as 100 per cent reliable truth I am going to find myself in difficulty. Similarly if I let my feelings eat away at things I know are actually true I'll hit problems. So, I know I am prepared for my talk at the next big conference I'm doing. But I am anxious, naturally, as my brain is drawing my attention to the fact that it is an important event. But if I misinterpret that anxiety as telling me I have some factual reason to be concerned, there's a very real risk that the anxiety itself may become the problem. This would be an emotional shortcut – instead of treating the emotion as a warning to look into something in more detail, I'd be treating it as truth.

When we are under stress, the unfortunate truth is that this kind of error becomes more and more likely – for two reasons. The first is that our brains, juggling many demands and struggling with fatigue, are forced to take exactly these kinds of shortcuts because they simply don't have the capacity to analyse everything at the same time. Some things therefore just have to be acted on without the sensible rational buffering that a bit of good thinking would give us. This is what happens when you are stressed out by something at work, or trying to get something finished, and your child comes to ask you a perfectly reasonable question. Without thinking you yell at them, annoyed with their unreasonable demands on you, interrupting you when you need to be able to think clearly. What your brain has done is assumed your emotion – irritation – was correct – meaning you treat them as though they are in the wrong. Then you realise all they were asking was when tea was going to be ready, and that it is very late and that you have totally lost track of time!

The second is to do with the strength and quality of our emotional responses. When we are under stress our emotional brains become more reactive in that our emotions can change more dramatically and swing up and down more suddenly. Hypervigilance (when your brain is on red alert) can add to this meaning that your brain triggers emotions for stimuli or situations it would normally ignore. Both of these mean that you are liable to be experiencing much more often the kind of strong emotions which would usually be fairly rare. In the event of such emotions – particularly anxiety or anger – your brain is much more prone to 'emotional hijack'.[2] This means that

---

2   Check out Chapter 3, 'Are you a stresshead?!' if you need a reminder about what emotional hijack is.

you act and react *before you think*, often responding dramatically, unpredictably and perhaps irrationally. This tendency becomes all the more acute when you are under pressure. Heard stories of people cracking in the moment and doing stupid things that they would never usually do? These things can very often be a sign of burnout.

In addition to leading to some bad choices and decisions, the main difficulty with this pattern of thinking is that it can very quickly lead to a downward spiral of emotional thinking. Your emotions are like a smoke alarm - they alert you to the *chance* of trouble ahead. If you assumed every time your smoke alarm went off that there was definitely a fire, you would be responding to a lot of false alarms! Treating your emotional responses as definitive truth is promoting them to a level in your brain at which they were never designed to operate. They need to be challenged, questioned, analysed, and often identified as false alarms. Without this, the world can feel a very difficult place, with anxieties, worries, frustrations and sadnesses around every corner. Add this perspective to an already stressed out brain and you can see how it doesn't lead anywhere good.

As with all areas of burnout the important thing is to recognise early warning signs of emotional exhaustion, and the things that signal that your brain is using emotional shortcuts in how it perceives the world. Watch out for emotions that come from nowhere, reactions that take you by surprise in hindsight. Be aware also of the thoughts that often accompany very emotional reasoning - fleeting thoughts of needing to escape, hit out, run away - things you would never normally even consider doing. These thoughts can be distressing but it is important not to ignore them or try to suppress them. Instead recognise them for what they are - a warning that you are near the emotional edge.

Are you on the brink?

Perhaps as you are reading this now you are aware of your own situation and the stress you are experiencing. How do you know if you have burned out, or if you are at risk? And what do you do if you are?

First steps - do not panic

Burnout is a very difficult place to be, and it is understandable why finding yourself there is so distressing. Most people who burn out have spent a very long time trying to keep an awful lot of things going without everything falling apart. Facing the fact that you cannot continue doing this for much longer is not easy and can trigger a lot of guilt. Remember that you don't have to just accept these feelings. Burnout is not a sign of weakness or any kind of failure, so do not use it to beat yourself up.

Remember that the most important thing in difficult times like these is to keep yourself safe. You may be finding that, particularly in moments of high pressure, you are fighting back thoughts which may be quite extreme or frightening. It is not unusual for people to find thoughts of suicide or of running away coming to mind – sometimes when they least expect them. Recognise these as what they are: a sign that your brain is under extreme pressure and is seeking a way out. They are an important warning that you need to slow down – and that you need help and support. Respond to them by getting that help.

The second most important – and perhaps the hardest – thing to do when you hit burnout is to *accept* where you are and manage the frustrations of your position. You will feel like you want to push through it, keep going, meet all the deadlines and pressures you have on you. You will not want to let people down and you may have worries about what will happen if you have to take time off work. Burnout is not something that anyone expected to find themselves dealing with. But in general the more you fight it the longer it will take you to recover and move on. Try to accept where you are and that you will need to take some time out to get back to normal.

Get some help and advice

The next thing to do if you are concerned is to head to your GP. It's quite likely that you are experiencing some worrying and/or distressing symptoms - physical or emotional. You might suspect that your symptoms are caused by stress - or you might be worried that they are something more, but there is only one way to find out for sure. Your GP will be able to check out your physical situation as well as get some insight into how you are doing emotionally. They'll also be able to help you take the first steps on the road to recovery.

Going to visit your GP isn't easy. In fact a lot of people say it is the hardest step to take. But in most cases the worst bit is worrying about it beforehand - it is usually a much better experience than you fear! If you can, try to see a GP who you know, and who you feel comfortable with. If you are having trouble arranging an appointment don't be afraid to explain a bit of what is going on to the receptionist, so that they understand why you want to see a particular doctor. You may be able to request a double appointment, so you don't feel under time pressure, or agree to come at a less busy time to see them. If you are finding it really hard you can bring a friend or family member with you. You could even write to the GP before the appointment (make sure the letter gets there a good few days before so s/he has time to read it) and explain a little of what you are going through in the letter.

Find some space to breathe

If you do feel under pressure, whether that is from work or due to other things going on in your life, you need to find some breathing space. Can you get some time away from those pressures? It's easy for us to feel like there's no way to escape from stress, but very often there are more possible solutions than we think. If you can't think of any, find a friend or family member you can chat to who might be able to help you think of some. Avoid the temptation to feel that you have to solve all your problems in one go in order for it to be helpful. Often just a couple of days away can give you a new perspective on what is going on. In more serious situations, where burnout has become much more difficult to handle, your GP might recommend that you take a longer time-out. This may mean signing you off work, or looking into some sources of support for other demands on you, such as family, etc. This is never easy - if you were good at stopping you probably wouldn't be where you are now! Think of it as a short term decision to help things get back on track long term. When you have time out, don't be tempted to use it to catch up on other things. Instead use it really effectively. Rest, relax and recuperate.[3]

Think about longer term

While you need to manage your frustration about not being able to carry on at your previous pace, there's nothing wrong with vowing not to get into this place again. Use your time out to put into place good things that will make it less likely to happen again: **routines** in terms of rest and time out; **rules** and boundaries concerning work and rest and **retraining,** to reduce the frequency of unhelpful thinking styles or anything that might be making you more prone to stress and anxiety.

Once you have had the chance to recharge your batteries a bit over the short term, you need to start to think about longer term changes. Are there things you might need to change? It is

---

3   Check out the first chapter in Part 2 - Chapter 7, 'Back to *basics*' - for more
    on this.

tempting to think of big changes – leaving your job or stepping down from positions of authority. It is, however, often worth considering smaller changes you could make instead. Very often it is not the big things we do, but the littler things we put pressure on ourselves to do *as well* which can push us over our limits. If you want to continue with some of the higher maintenance things in your life, perhaps there are some simpler things you can share, or find other ways to do. Remember you are not super(wo)man. There is nothing wrong with accepting that you have limits. It may be that something as simple as doing your shopping on the internet instead of going to the supermarket, or arranging a childcare rota with a friend so you don't end up trying to juggle your kids *and* that thing it is almost impossible to do with them around, or getting a cleaner a few hours a week, or sometimes not making it to the gym 5 times every week, or maybe just doing a short run instead of the full length one … whoever you are and whatever your schedule challenges I am willing to bet there are small changes you could make which could take a surprising amount of pressure off. Think about keeping a diary for a few days of what exactly you do each hour of each day. What are the little things that push you over the edge – the things you don't really have time for but you have to do anyway or you feel guilty?

As well as thinking about changes you might need to make to the way you spend your time, there are some other key issues that you are likely to find it helpful to think through. These will be the focus of Part 2 of this book as we think about how to fuel and refuel your way through whatever life throws at you in the future.

Over to you ...

Thinking about whether you might be close to burnout RIGHT NOW – where do you think you are NOW on the following lines?

PHYSICALLY

Plenty of energy. Feel lively, vibrant and 'up' for most things

Feel tired and unmotivated most of the time. Exhausted.

INTELECTUALLY/COGNITIVELY

Creative, sharp, find it easy to come up with new ideas. Enthusiastic and happy to be involved in things

Cynical. Out of ideas. Find it hard to be optimistic that an idea will work anyway. Very uninspired.

EMOTIONALLY

Feel flat or low a lot of the time. Emotionally volatile – prone to feeling really angry or sad without much provocation.

Optimistic, patient, feel generally positive and bright.

SOCIALLY

| Engaged and involved with the lives of others. Find it easy to empathise and feel sympathy for others. Connecting regularly and easily with friends and family | Withdrawn, avoiding contact with others. Feel increasingly isolated from friends and family. Find it hard to communicate with others or to care what they are feeling |

SPIRITUALLY

| Find it easy to spend time with God and to pray. Worship comes easily, feel very connected with God and the Holy Spirit in all areas of life | Struggle to find time and/or energy to spend time with God. Worship difficult or other things get in the way. Feel a sense of loss of meaning or purpose. God feels distant and/or irrelevant. |

Have you (or anyone close to you) noticed any other symptoms that you think might be because you are close to burnout?

Have you noticed any changes in how you feel about things you usually enjoy; e.g. not wanting to do them, finding they do not bring you pleasure or even cause stress?

Are you experiencing any strong emotional reactions which might be related to your stress levels?

If you do feel on the brink of burnout …

Remember: Don't panic. But do act. Your first step is to get some help and advice – your GP is the best first person to talk to. Do you need to share how you are feeling with someone to ask them to help you make an appointment? If so, write down who you are going to talk to, and when (be specific!). Tick it off once you have asked them for their help.

Now you need to call and make an appointment with your GP. Remember it might be best to call at a quiet time of day. Note down here the date and time of your appointment here.

Another good thing to do is to schedule in some time where you can find some space to breathe and rest. RIGHT NOW, can you think of a day you can take COMPLETELY OFF from your main pressures? Can you plan somewhere to go that day, or how you are going to spend it? Write down your plans here:

It's also a good idea to think about how you can make some space in your calendar over the next month or so. Is there something you can step back from for a time to get some extra rest? Think about what you could take a break from and write it down here:

PART 2

7

Back to *basics*

Part 2 of this book is all about practical solutions to help you manage stress – to deal with high stress situations and keep going when things get crazy. The best place to start is to go back to basics. What are your core needs as a human being, the way you were designed?

To do this I'm going to look at the clearest depiction of stress and burnout in the Bible – coming from the life of Elijah.

About Elijah ...

Elijah was a prophet living in the ninth century before Jesus. The section of his life story which I want to consider falls in 1 Kings 19, but to understand the context it's good to start with 1 Kings 18. To set the background, the story occurs in the midst of a time when the Kingdom of Israel was being ruled by foreign kings.

The King at this time was a man called Ahab. Ahab wasn't a great king – amongst other things, he allowed the worship of other Gods, including Baal, the ancient Canaan God of rain, thunder and lightning. Ahab's wife, Jezebel, was actually a priestess of this religion. Elijah is sent into the story in 1 Kings 17, to tell the King that because of his actions there will be a severe drought in the country which will go on for years. Elijah is kept safe by God through the three years of drought which follow, during which Jezebel keeps busy by hunting down and killing God's prophets. Eventually Elijah is the only prophet left.

It all comes to a dramatic showdown. God tells Elijah to go direct to King Ahab, and that he, God, will send rain. The resulting meeting takes place on the top of Mount Carmel: Ahab and Elijah, together with the (numerous) prophets of Baal. It culminates in a dramatic contest as Elijah challenges the prophets of Baal to make fire (well worth a read in 1 Kings 18:16-46). The prophets of Baal come to a sticky end and the chapter closes with an almighty rainstorm just as God had promised.

It's what happens next in 1 Kings 19 which is so interesting for our purposes. Elijah is hot on the heels of victory – he has pulled off an amazing miracle and done it in front of a huge audience. Obeying God, he had taken what must have felt like a huge risk, walking right up to the very person who was trying to kill him and challenging him with what he was doing wrong – and it paid off! He stood up to not just one person but to a crowd of jeering, challenging prophets of a strange and quite sinister religion. It has all gone remarkably well! But it has taken its impact. A message comes from Jezebel – a furious letter, threatening his life. And Elijah crumples. There is no other word for it. This amazing man who has stood apparently calm in front of hundreds of chanting, bleeding, shrieking prophets of Baal is totally floored by … a letter. He seems to have a kind of emotional collapse. The Bible tells us he was '*afraid, and ran for his life*' (1 Kings 19:3, NIV). He journeys into the wilderness and then lies under a tree. 'I have had enough Lord,' he prays 'Take my life; I am no better than my ancestors' (1 Kings 19:4).

This whole tale reminds me so much of the many stories I have heard about people who have suffered stress-related breakdowns. They have typically been people I know who manage huge responsibility and strain in their jobs, but a final straw that might otherwise seem minor or insignificant seems to push them over the edge. Elijah had thought the worst was over, so to get that letter was just too much. He was pushed beyond his limits.

In this situation, God's response is very interesting. You won't see a lecture, a 'get a grip' pep talk, or a telling off. God doesn't advise a long course of therapy or medication (not that these are bad things in the right situations), nor does he send someone to pray for Elijah, lay on hands or anoint him with oil. What God, who created our human body and brains, did for this particular battered, exhausted, burned out specimen, tells us a lot about three vital basic needs we all have even today.

1. Sleep

God's first action is to do … well apparently nothing! What he does is *lets Elijah sleep*. The other things which he needed came later. Sleep, it seems is a central, crucial, inescapable part of being human. And too little for too long can have a huge impact on our ability to deal with stress.

In the beginning …

If we're going back to basics and think about sleep, it is good to go right back to the beginning in thinking about the way we were designed. Genesis kicks off by telling the amazing story of how we – and the world – were made. I was once out on a trip looking for a new book for my daughter. I was flicking through the pages of lots of children's books when I came across one which was all about how the world came about. It was a fantastic book, full of bright coloured pages. I was loving it as I flicked through – and then I came to the very first page. It had a huge picture of space, black and empty. Written across the page in great big white letters were these words;

'IN THE BEGINNING THERE WAS … NOTHING.'

The Bible tells us a very important fact that differs from these scientific explanations, filling in a very significant 'gap'. It tells us that 'In the beginning, GOD …' (Genesis 1:1, NIV). Whatever you believe about what happened next, whatever science can teach us, it all began with God. Not random, not chance, not chaos, but God.

Genesis carries on to outline how God began to create order in our universe. We see light finally shine through, then the separation of the heavens and the earth; the development of islands, the sun and moon and finally – life. Beginning with fish and birds, the earth begins to see living things. And then, last but certainly not least, God creates something amazing: humans.

We're not given a lot of detail about the creation of all those animals, bird and fish. The Bible doesn't tell us what God was thinking when he made giraffes, why he bothered to make wasps or what was going on with all those weird and wonderful fish that live so deep in the ocean we're only just starting to understand their complexity. But it does give some more, very key information about us humans. 'Then God said, "Let us make mankind in our image, in our likeness"' (Genesis 1:26, NIV). Humans, unlike anything else in all creation, were created in God's likeness. *The Message* puts it beautifully: 'God spoke: "Let us make human beings in our image, make them *reflecting our nature*"' (Genesis 1:26, *The Message*, italics mine).

Understanding this is key to appreciating some of the things inbuilt into our human bodies which we sometimes find frustrating. These set the parameters of what we need to survive – and more than that, to *thrive*. And one of those elements is a very basic rhythm that needs to be built into our lives. We can see it explained in Genesis 2:1: 'By the seventh day God had finished the work he had been doing; so on the seventh day he rested from all his work.' (Gen 2:1, NIV). God demonstrates this foundation level rhythm, which is echoed not just in us but in all creation. It's about the balance between two things: *work* and *rest*. Both are important, and both are distinct. There is a period of *work*, but it is followed by a deliberate and significant period of *rest*.

We, just like God, are designed to live by a rhythm of these two things: work and rest. Both are essential to us. In our modern 24/7 world, we are very prone to neglecting our rest. We are also at risk of simply blurring the boundaries between the two so that we struggle after a while to recognise the two clear categories. But in the beginning the distinction was clear.

Running on empty
Elijah had faced a situation where he had done a tremendous amount of work. He had had such a crazy few days, I'm guessing he hadn't had much time to rest. Then he had run all the way from Mount Carmel first to a place called Jezreel and then finally on to Beersheba in Judah. This is a long way - around 180km to be precise. Google Maps suggests I could do it in a car in about 2 hours but running would have taken a lot longer! Elijah must have been done in! What is interesting though is how much of his stress reaction was tied up in his exhaustion. This probably explains a lot about how he reacted to Jezebel's message - and the amazing contrast between the man who stood so bravely and defiantly on Mount Carmel and the man who fled and ran all the way to where God finds him. Elijah has become so exhausted he is showing many of the signs of burnout. Before he sleeps he cannot even face living. He does not have the energy for that most basic of things - existing. He feels he cannot carry on any more.

God's initial response is very interesting. After all, Elijah had just expressed a wish to die - quite a dramatic request. You might expect some kind of dialogue, even if it was of the 'It's not really that bad' category. But instead, God doesn't even try to have a conversation with him. Elijah was so exhausted he just wasn't able to think straight. This is a useful thing to note: when we are exhausted, sometimes our thinking can go haywire. Emotions can lurch dramatically and thoughts which we would otherwise never entertain can feel rational and true. We need to recognise that there can be times when our thinking and our emotions might *not be reliable*. These are not times to make big decisions. It may genuinely not be as bad as it feels! What we need – urgently – is some rest.

Elijah, just like you and me, was a human created in the image of God. He needed regular rest in order to function well. Have you ever noticed just how much harder life is when you are tired? It is one of the cruellest ironies of having a small baby that if there was ever a time in your life when you needed to be feeling at your strongest emotionally, sleep deprivation means you spend much of your time on the edge of emotional chaos. Anyone who has ever done shift work, or had to pull an all-nighter to get through exams or college work will know how hard that is. Some people, struggling on with severe insomnia, wade through life in the swampy muddy mess that is feeling totally worn out. I've often heard people joke 'sleep is for wimps' – but the truth is sleep is for *humans*! Even Jesus – God in a human body – was at times overwhelmed with this all too human need to rest.

If you are dealing with stress, or living/working in a high stress environment, getting good sleep is really important. Now I know what you are going to say – you can't. Maybe you have children who keep you awake, or conditions which mean you find it hard to sleep, partners who snore or dogs that bark. But it is *so* important that you sleep. Make it a priority. Whether that means visiting the doctor for advice on how to sleep better, taking turns to be responsible for children who are up in the night, sleeping in the spare room – do it. This single action will give you immense help in managing stress.

A word about prayer and healing

Take a moment with me to think about exactly how Elijah recovers from his breakdown. He is in direct communication with God – and yet, he is not instantly healed. Instead it is through a very human and natural process that he recovers. Even then though it is not immediate. After Elijah sleeps he feels a bit better – enough at first to eat and drink – but then he needs to sleep again. Eventually he does feel well enough to journey to connect with God – but note that it takes a few good sleeps before he gets to this place. There is no 'instant fix'. It takes time.

It is natural when someone is in a place of emotional or physical breakdown that people want to pray for them – and it is a very good thing to do. After all, what really gets Elijah back on track emotionally is his meeting with God – that time to connect and refuel spiritually. But we must recognise that what people often need at first in order to recover is time – time to rest, sleep and eat and drink healthily. This doesn't mean God isn't 'in' that time, but we must remember that God has created our bodies with certain needs. God is unlikely to heal us in order that we can circumvent these basic needs!

Too often there can be a pressure on people to 'be better' almost instantly after prayer. Prayer is very important for people who are in the midst of burnout – but so are practical things that help them to rest and recuperate. And we must make sure that we do not put pressure on them to recovery quickly, but recognise that it may take time, and that no matter how frustrating we might find it, that is very much part of God's design.

2. Eat

The next step God leads Elijah through is one of physical refuelling. He gets him to eat and drink. Now, from what the Bible tells us this isn't anything special – it's no three course meal, no Michelin stars. But after a very stressful time it sounds pretty good: fresh bread and some water. Your body's need for physical fuel is fairly. If you have been burning the candle at both ends, you may well need to refuel with what you eat.

I know what you're thinking here – that you eat plenty already! But the trouble with stress is that it changes the kind of thing we eat, so that we crave high sugar snacks. This is because of the impact stress has on your blood sugar, raising it and draining your reserves. Thanks to the influence of cortisol, it also makes us more prone to laying down fat stores in precisely the places that are least healthy – around our organs and middles. Actually what you need in order to recover from stress, or to manage it well, is good, nourishing food that releases energy slowly into your bloodstream and provides you with the building blocks you need for cell repair and to keep you healthy. Stress tends to leave us relying on precisely the kinds of foods that in the long term leave us not just at risk of gaining weight, but also lacking in key nutrients and vitamins.

A lot of the problems surrounding what we eat when we are stressed stem from how difficult it can be to sit down and actually eat a proper meal. Stress eating tends to involve a lot more snacking, grazing, or grabbing things 'on the run.' This is more likely the more tired you get – brain imaging shows that the brains of people who are sleep deprived have a much greater response to pictures of 'junk' food. In fact the area of their brain that 'lights up' is the same one which responds when addicts are shown pictures of their drug! We also know that the levels of certain hormones in your blood which control appetite rise when you are sleep deprived, making you crave food. So lack of sleep and that 'constant grazing' behaviour really do go together – and the chances are this leaves you eating rubbish all day and never actually stopping to have a proper nutritious meal.

Perhaps you feel like it's to be expected that you eat less healthily when you are under stress – we've all heard about 'comfort' eating. Studies show some people certainly do eat more under times of pressure or high anxiety. But they also reveal that this does little to lift mood. It actually often causes us to feel *worse* in the long term. So although you might *think* that tub of ice cream will make you feel better, it probably won't. Particularly in times of stress, healthy eating is important – even if what you really feel like is a large coffee and a pastry.

Whilst we're talking about coffee, let's think about caffeine. It's a classic 'pick me up' in times of stress, and can help us concentrate and improve attention. But did you know that caffeine also affects the way you metabolise or deal with food and sugar? It makes your body a little bit less good at using insulin to deal with the sugar in your blood, keeping it more raised – which might keep you energised in the short term but isn't a great idea in the long term. Caffeine also has other effects which can actually make you *more* stressed, reducing the quality (and often quantity) of sleep, making you more prone to anxiety and tension and making physical symptoms of that – such as feeling shaky or your heart racing – more likely. Perhaps the trickiest thing is that caffeine really is addictive. Once your body gets used to it, it takes a higher dose to get the same effect. And people who are used to drinking a lot of caffeine actually show surprisingly little response from it.

I have already mentioned my theory that a lot of people who are classic 'introverts' use caffeine in order to help them function well in more 'extrovert' contexts and communication styles. It helps them match that more extrovert style of communication. Beware if that is you – the combination of the stressful environment plus the potential for overconsumption of caffeine could have a bigger impact on you than you think. Caffeine really is something best enjoyed in small doses. You don't need to avoid it completely, but be wary of how (and how often) you use it.

3. Time to connect with God

The first two of Elijah's basic needs were physical. The third focuses on a different, but equally important need – his spiritual health. This may seem surprising. After all, Elijah has just been hearing from God – he's clearly a man spiritual enough to be the main player in a significant miracle. But in a crucial way he has become disconnected from God. It's something to do with the difference between our personal connection with God and our spending time serving God.

Those of us with older children will recognise all too well what happens after they have spent the whole day together at school. They get in – and straight away they're longing to go on Facebook, or to FaceTime, to text or to call their friends. Sometimes you can have spent all day with someone but still not have really connected with them. This is where Elijah is, and it is often the same for many people working and volunteering in the church.

When the Bible talks about someone being 'filled', it's noticeable that it refers to two different kinds of filling. One is very much a permanent 'background' filling. So, Jesus is *'filled with wisdom'* (Luke 2:40, NIV) and 'full of the Holy Spirit' (Luke 4:1, NIV), not just in those moments but all the time. But there is also a kind of 'in the moment' filling – a spiritual burst or flare which fills people right when and where they need it. So, the disciples are *'filled with the Holy Spirit.'* at Pentecost (Acts 2:4) – and there are many other examples where this kind of spirit 'rush' occurs (for example Peter in Acts 4:8). It is essential we remain connected with God, and able to experience these bursts of spiritual wisdom and energy. If we fail to, relying on our 'background' filling, we may find that it slowly ebbs away.

Maybe you feel like you spend enough time with God as it is – you can never seem to get away from the church building! Maybe the last thing you feel like doing on your precious day or evening off is praying. But as a human you have a basic need to be continually reconnecting with God, refilling and refuelling with God's spirit. Think of it a bit like plugging in your phone. This is not physical refuelling – it is spiritual refuelling – but it is just as essential – especially if you are pushing the limits, living a hectic, busy, stressful, God-serving life.

Jesus shared a unique relationship with God the Father, as his son – but in spite of this, he knew the limitations of being human. So what did he do? He made regular time to 'refuel' his connection with God. The gospels are peppered with examples of when Jesus stopped to pray – particularly when things were very busy or stressful or when there was a significant decision to be made. So, Jesus prayed after a hectic time in Capernum where he had taught, and healed many people (Mark 1:35); when crowds of people were turning up every day to be healed and to hear him speak (Luke 5:16); before choosing his disciples (Luke 6:12); after feeding 5000 people and pondering what to tell his disciples about who he really was (Luke 9:18); before teaching the disciples how to pray (Luke 11:1); and of course in Gethsemane when he knew the very next day he would be betrayed and led to his death (26:36-43).

Journey
What is noticeable in each of these circumstances is not just that Jesus prayed, but that in order to do so, he had to make a particular decision to pray, and then seek somewhere quiet and private in order to focus properly. Elijah had to journey considerably before he was ready to connect with God. Sometimes in stress-filled times our minds are buzzing so much it is nearly impossible to hear God speak, or feel God with us. We need to take steps to travel somewhere calmer in order to connect with God properly (more on this in the next chapter). Elijah journeyed for 40 days and 40 nights - this symbolic time frame which we see in other parts of the Bible. It may not refer to a literal 40 days - this number was often used to signify a general period of time rather than the precise number - but what we know is that Elijah journeyed for a long time.

Here again is the warning not to rush things. Elijah had a *considerable* break before he reconnected with God and got back on his ministry 'train'. If you have been hit with a very stressful time, remember that you need to recover not just physically but emotionally and spiritually as well, and this takes time. Sometimes you need to focus on the basics for a while before you are ready to begin to heal spiritually. We must avoid putting pressure on ourselves and becoming frustrated at our apparent lack of spiritual connection and trust God's own timescale for our healing.

So, Elijah travelled both literally and emotionally in order to be able to connect with God. But how and where did he do this, and what changed so that he was able to communicate effectively with God? To understand that, we need to move on to the next chapter and think about another essential need we all have: calm.

Over to you ...

Take a moment to think about the three key areas covered in this chapter.

Sleep

Are you getting enough sleep? What's your instinctive response to this question?

To help you think more about your sleep, here are some more questions to ponder:

How many hours do you actually spend in bed? Lots of people don't sleep enough because they just don't make enough time for sleep, or because they get distracted and end up doing other things when they should be going to bed. Is this you?

Is there anything waking you up or making you sleep less soundly? (This might include worries, bad dreams, snoring partners, children, etc.)

Do you give yourself time to wind down before trying to go to sleep? Very few people can turn off their brains just like that - are you expecting your brain to go from 100 to 0 in one step? Do you do things (e.g. work) before going to bed that wind your brain *up* instead of *down*?

Do you use 'blue light' emitting devices (e.g. iPhones, iPad, other smartphones, etc.) in the hour before you try to go to sleep? (This has been linked with problems falling asleep.) If so, is this something you could try to change - and see if it has any effect?

Do you have any problems with sleep that you need to talk to your doctor about?

What do YOU need to change so that you meet your basic need for sleep better?

1

2

3

Eating/Diet

In general how healthily would you say you eat?

Do you generally get your 'five a day'?

Do you have times when you eat not because of hunger but because of something else (e.g. feeling bored, sad or angry)?

Do you eat a lot of sugary food to keep your energy levels up through the day?

Do you ever skip meals due to busy-ness, dieting or not feeling hungry due to stress?

Do you monitor what you eat? If so, is this a helpful thing (some people monitor in order to eat less fat, or to keep to a diet for a health condition) or a difficult thing (some people find they obsess about food and find it hard to let themselves eat without feeling guilt and/or calorie counting)?

Do you have any problems with eating which you need to talk to your doctor about?

What do you need to change about your eating patterns in order to better meet your basic need for food?

1

2

3

Connecting with God

Do you have a regular time each day when you stop to pray and/or read the Bible?

Do you properly connect with God or do you sometimes just 'go through the motions'?

What do you find hardest about connecting with God during times of stress?

When you have time, what things inspire you and help you connect with God?

What do you need to change about how you connect with God in order to better meet this basic need?

1

2

3

8

Keep *calm!*

Having taken some time to look at the history of our own creation, and to understand the importance of a basic rhythm of work and rest, I want to think more about our spiritual lives and how the craziness of the pace of twenty-first-century life can sometimes interrupt that. We've seen how Elijah had to journey to find a space where he could connect with God. But *how* exactly did he connect with God?[1]

Once his journey was over, Elijah found a cave and went to sleep there overnight. It was then that God spoke to him, asking him what he was doing there. He replies at once with a heartfelt wail of complaint about his situation. It only needs 'It's not fair!' to sound like a proper teenage rant! This shows just how beyond his limits Elijah was – just like a teenager experiencing emotions they don't know how to deal with, he is buckling under stress he cannot handle any more.

What happens next, to my mind, is full of drama and great scenery. God tells him to go out and stand on the mountain, because he, God, is going to pass by. Three things happen – all of them loud and wild. They are just the sort of things we probably expect when God turns up. First there is a wind so powerful it 'tore mountains apart and shattered the rocks' (1 Kings 19:11,

---

1 You can follow the story as it continues in 1 Kings 19:9-13.

NIV) – but it turns out 'the Lord was not in the wind.' Next
came an earthquake – but God wasn't in that either. Finally a fire
came – but no sign of God.

We often expect God to appear with great drama and
significance, in scenes full of trumpet sounds and amazing scenes.
How often, when we want to connect with God, do we look
in places which are loud and full of busy-ness? But we may well
fail to find God in those things. In fact, even if God were there,
how easy it would be to miss God in the drama of the moment.
When we are stressed – in times of real pressure and mayhem –
our yearning for God can be magnified by our apparent failure
to find God in those places and our frustration as our desperate
need to connect with God goes unmet day after day. Running
on spiritual empty is a very difficult way to live, particularly if
you are under a lot of pressure. What we need to realise is that
we may be looking for God in the wrong places, and failing to
journey to where we need to be to meet with God. Because
actually, in Elijah's story, God is in what *follows* the drama – in a
gentle whisper.

It's taken me years – decades in fact – to learn how quietly
God can act. Have you ever had an experience like I did the
other day? I was busy trying to make dinner, and also to do a
host of other things because I knew that as soon as I had got the
children to bed I had a meeting to go to. It was manic, busy , hot,
pots were boiling over, food was burning, the radio was on – I
was multitasking like a mad person. It took ages for me to 'tune
in' to the sounds of my son who, it turns out, had been standing
next to me asking me something for ages. That time it was just
a small boy with a question, but when I think of that moment it
makes me think of how many times I may have failed to hear the
small voice of God in the midst of my crazy, busy days.

Mind full?

Mindfulness has had a bad press in Christian circles at times, but actually it is often misunderstood. Mindfulness speaks of the opposite of what I have just described – of being in tune and in control of where our mind is going so that we do not become overwhelmed by chaos and noise and as a result miss quieter, more subtle calls on our attention. Being 'mindful' of something therefore speaks of a decision to turn our attention to it. You can see an example in Psalm 8:4: 'When I consider your heavens, the work of your fingers, the moon and the stars, which you have set in place, what is mankind that you are mindful of them, human beings that you care for them?' (NIV). This great psalm of worship starts by talking about the amazing complexity of the world, the earth and the heavens. And then comes this verse – it wonders how, with all that going on, God is 'mindful', i.e. chooses to turn God's mind – to humans.

Mindfulness teaches techniques and skills which enable us to start to overcome a risk that we might be so preoccupied with all the myriad of things our brains are coordinating that we miss less demanding but vital things. One example of these is our emotions. Psychologists have identified a group of people who have become so disconnected from their own emotions that they almost seem unable to describe or identify them – they are 'alexithymic' (literally a 'lack of words' for emotions). Of course they do experience emotions – one theory is that they have become so good at suppressing or ignoring them that they have become almost unaware of them. In their busy minds, emotions – especially negative emotions – go un-noticed, but the impact they have are often all too apparent: high scorers on measures of alexithymia are at greater risk of various psychological and mental health problems. Mindfulness skills – often used now in conjunction with therapies like CBT – help people connect with their own thoughts and feelings again.

Mindfulness is also an important concept for us as spiritual people because failing to be 'mindful' in our day to day life runs a very real risk that we will miss the '*still small voice*' (1 Kings 19:12, KJV) of God. When we are stressed or overloaded the irony is that the very thing which causes us to be in greater need of hearing from God may render us unable to perceive God's voice.

I remember years ago going walking with my husband in the dales in Yorkshire. We were in the middle of an amazing landscape, green and totally deserted as far as the eye could see. Then far in the distance we heard and saw a tractor pull up and a man climbed out. He stood by the tractor, took a whistle from his pocket and blew it three times. Then he leaned back on the tractor and waited. We were baffled - the silence of the dales seemed undisturbed by his actions and we could still see nothing and no one in any direction. But then, after a few minutes, a sheep appeared, leaping over the horizon. Then another - then another - and within minutes the whole area was full of sheep of all shapes, sizes and colours, running towards the tractor. It was pretty impressive! Clearly this had been their call - for food I suppose - and they heard it from miles away. In an instant it interrupted whatever they were doing (not that sheep lead particularly busy lives!) and they responded instinctively and immediately.

It made me think of how we hear God. 'My sheep hear my voice, and I know them, and they follow me,' said Jesus (John 10:27 RSV) - some translations (e.g. *The Message*) say 'my sheep *recognise* my voice' (my italics). This is what mindfulness can teach us - how to ensure we are in a place where we will recognise and hear God's voice so that we can respond, regardless of what we are in the middle of at the time. Mindfulness teaches us how to 'tune in'. It is about re-learning to pay attention - to notice the little messages, whether they are from our bodies or our minds, or perhaps that still small voice of God. Mindfulness encourages us to learn to stop and take a moment of calm to focus – but also it teaches us to be better focused even in times when all around us is chaos.

How to be mindful …

You can practise mindfulness in various ways, and there are several excellent books written about it[2] – but here's a short exercise to try. This is a classic mindfulness practice linked to the way you eat – something we can all too easily do 'mind-less-ly'. Do you ever find, particularly if you are eating at your desk or are doing something, that you sit down with your lunch and before you know it is gone and you didn't even notice eating it? That is 'mind-less' eating! This exercise challenges you to take a few minutes out to eat something – popularly a raisin but I often get people to do this exercise with a Malteser instead.

In order to mindfully eat your Malteser, you want to focus your mind as entirely as you can on the whole experience. Instead of just throwing it into your mouth and chomping, really consider it. Before you even put it in your mouth, take a moment to 'experience' it with your other senses. What does it feel like? Can you feel the chocolate melting a bit in your fingers? Can you smell it? And look at it – really look – notice little imperfections in the chocolate.

Next pop it in your mouth. Note the way your body responds to the chocolate – your mouth starting to water, the feel of it on your tongue, the different taste tensions (is your mouth watering even now as you are reading this?!). Crunch or suck the Malteser – up to you, but as you do so take your time and really notice the different sensations as you eat – the texture of it against your tongue, the taste, the way it dissolves in your mouth. Notice the way it feels as you swallow it and the change in the taste as it leaves your mouth and gradually becomes a memory.

---

2 See Appendix 1 for ideas for more reading on this and all the topics raised in this book.

Mindfully eating Maltesers may seem like a bit of fun, but it introduces a way of experiencing things which may require a big adjustment of our minds. Instead of doing one thing with our mind meanwhile on one hundred other things, it encourages us to focus on what we are doing, and connect with our own, often ignored, bodies. It contradicts a move in our culture right now to never fully focus on anything and to be almost continually distracted. Think about it – the last time you had to wait for a train or a bus, or in a supermarket queue, what did you do? An awful lot of us will have grabbed our smartphones, checked messages, read Twitter or tweeted something. Mindfulness encourages us to take advantage of moments we have - not to distract ourselves with other things but to *experience* the world and life in all its fullness.

You can practice mindfulness in lots of other ways - and you can certainly include it as part of your prayer life. Try going out into nature for your next prayer time. Grab a seat somewhere peaceful and for a moment, just sit. I like to start by sitting in silence and trying to identify every single sound I can hear, one at a time. It really helps to focus my brain on the time and place rather than all the thoughts buzzing around it. You'll be surprised at how you gradually tune in to sounds you never heard before. Then perhaps read a passage of scripture about God's creation - maybe Genesis 1, or something really praise-filled like Psalm 8. Then look around you at all the nature surrounding you - really take a moment to revel in the reality of the example of God's creation all around you. Another great thing to do is to take a 'mindful' walk – again, instead of 'just' walking, really listen, experience with all your senses that walk and the world around you as you go. If it is warm enough even take your shoes off so you can feel the ground beneath your feet.

Post burnout, or in times of stress, mindfulness practices can really help you to reconnect with God. Don't be alarmed if at first your usual practices seem to leave you feeling 'cold'. Think about taking time out, like Jesus did and journey somewhere

specifically to pray. Very often the distance between this place
and your everyday life helps you to 'find' your spiritual self.
What you do or where you go is up to you – be creative and
explore lots of things. Think about surrounding yourself with
nature and the brilliance of creation – long walks or bike rides
in the country, or time spent late in an evening gazing up at the
night sky. Take time to experience the creativity of great music
or art. Experiment with silence – or with sounds. Some people
prefer solitude, others find it easier to be lost in a crowd of
people worshipping. Don't feel pressure to fit into what works
for other people, or for everything you try to be helpful. Instead
find what works for you.

Once your mind is focused, and some of the everyday 'chatter'
in your brain is paused for a moment, you will become so much
better focused, and in a great place to talk – and of course to
listen – to God. Practising calm in this way can be an invaluable
antidote to stress – like using a fire extinguisher on the fraught
bits of our brains. Have you been seeking God for days? Weeks?
Months? If you feel like you have been crying out for days and
feel like you are getting no response, try taking some time out to
seek and find calm. You may find yourself suddenly able to hear
what God has been saying all along.

Drink it in

Moments of calm can be oases in the desert that is stress. Managing
to press 'pause' on the pace of life just for small moments like
this helps us find ourselves, and find time to connect with God,
improving how well we respond and our capacity to manage
difficult times. The need for these moments is inbuilt into who
we are. Ever heard the phrase 'Stop the world, I want to get off'?
If you are feeling like this, practicing finding calm may well help.
In fact, learning how to find calm in the middle of chaos is a key
step in improving how you manage stress.

By the way …

Before we move on from Elijah's story, there's one last thing I want to mention. Spending time with God helped Elijah, but in this case God did set in motion one practical change as well to avoid Elijah getting this exhausted in future: he introduced to him the man who would eventually succeed him as the Lord's prophet but who for now became … his assistant! (see 1 Kings 19:19-21). Learning to manage stress better is all very well but sometimes we do need to take practical steps and recognise that we cannot do it all on our own!

Over to you ...

Have you had a chance to practice a mindfulness exercise yet? If not then do it now – try mindfully eating a Malteser. (Or something like a raisin if you don't have any sweets!)

How did you find this task?

Do you think you have a tendency to do things 'on automatic pilot' when you are stressed?

What do you think happens to your own feelings, emotions and thoughts in those times?

Do you ever have trouble concentrating or doing things like falling asleep because your mind is 'racing' or still focused on something else?

Psalm 23:2-3 says 'He lets me rest in green meadows; he leads me beside peaceful streams. He renews my strength.' When did you last experience a real moment of calm and tranquility?

9

Chill out! How to get better at relaxing

So, you know that resting is important; you've taken on board the value of moments of mindfulness and you understand why calm is such an important part of your week. The only trouble is how on earth to fit it in!

Relaxation can feel like the least of your problems when life has gone crazy and your stress levels are at the max. 'If only I had the time!' you might be thinking, or 'Chance would be a fine thing'. We tend to treat relaxation as something we do once everything else is done – it's that thing we do on holidays or perhaps on Christmas Day after we've eaten too much at lunch. The rest of the time, it isn't something that comes easily. A recent study found that many people find themselves feeling guilty if they spend any significant time relaxing in the average week. We talk about 'guilty pleasures' but for some of us anything that doesn't involve being productive is exactly that – and as a result it's something we do very rarely, as a special treat or on a special occasion.

The problem with this attitude is that relaxation is part of this great work-rest cycle which is a central feature of the design structure of our bodies. If we never learn to incorporate it into the regular rhythm of our life, we are very likely to start to find ourselves struggling with problems due to stress. But very few of us do learn to include relaxation in our schedules. In fact many people don't realise relaxation is something they have to learn at all. The most common response I get when I talk to people about relaxation is something like 'oh, I'm not much good at that,' or 'I'm just not that kind of person'. But the truth is that *all people* need to relax – and not just on special occasions – *regularly*. Although admittedly some personality types find relaxation easier than others, it is something we all need to learn to do.

The most important part of your week

Relaxation is important for everyone. But if we start to consider people who are experiencing times of stress, or who tend to place themselves under pressure, it becomes even more essential. Relaxation is the antidote to stress. Periods of relaxation balance out the times of stress in your life and keep you stable.

Right from the start we can see the importance of times of rest and relaxation reflected in the Bible – most notably in the laws that God gave to his people. In the midst of the commandments, alongside instructions not to murder or worship any other Gods, we see this:

> 'Remember the Sabbath day by keeping it holy. Six days
> you shall labor and do all your work, but the seventh day
> is a Sabbath to the Lord your God. On it you shall not
> do any work, neither you, nor your son or daughter, nor
> your male or female servant, nor your animals, nor any
> foreigner residing in your towns. For in six days the Lord
> made the heavens and the earth, the sea, and all that is
> in them, but he rested on the seventh day. Therefore the
> Lord blessed the Sabbath day and made it holy'
> (Exodus 20:8-11, NIV).

The priority of this commandment is demonstrated in its position in the list of commandments – fourth out of the ten. That's before 'You shall not murder', before 'Honour your father and mother', before 'You shall not steal.' It is *important!* And yet although most of us would not think of breaking these other commandments, we probably break this one more regularly than any.

It seems that God was aware from the start of how tricky a commandment this one would be, and the high likelihood that the people would slip up. In fact, there had already been examples of this: God provided food for the Israelites with manna in the desert. They were commanded not to collect manna on the seventh day – but still some people did go out and try (Exodus 16:27). God reminds people again and again of this commandment. And each reminder offers further information about why the Sabbath laws are so important. So, straight after the commandments are given, when more detailed laws to cover various circumstances are given, the Sabbath laws are expanded and it is made clear they apply to more than just the people – even farming must follow a Sabbath pattern (Exodus 23:10-11). As for the people, the purpose of the Sabbath and the command not to work on that day is explained as being 'so that your ox and your donkey may rest, and so that the slave born in your household and the foreigner living among you may be refreshed' (Exodus 23:12, NIV). Here then lies that sense of humans and animals needing the rest and relaxation that the Sabbath brings in order to refresh them. But it is more than refreshing – the Hebrew word used here literally talks about a new soul – the result of the Sabbath, when kept, is a *complete renewal of your soul - your inner being*. Resting and taking regular time out to relax and focus on God restores us to where we were before our stresses hit.

It's easy when you look at the instructions in Exodus regarding the Sabbath to see why it might be particularly important in times of hard work and stress. But we wrestle with an all too human tendency to skip it particularly in those times. And you can see God's awareness of this risk in Exodus 31 – after delivering a very complex and detailed list of instructions and works needed to build the tabernacle, altar, etc., God issues a clear warning: 'You *must* observe my Sabbaths' (Exodus 31:13, NIV, my italics). Clearly God was aware of the risk that with so much work to do the Sabbath might get pushed out. The message is emphasised again in Exodus 34 when God outlines the nature of the covenant he is making with the people. Once again they are reminded that on the seventh day they must rest, but this time another note is added: 'even during the ploughing season and harvest you must rest' (v.21, NIV).

The message here then is clear. Rest and relaxation is a vital, central part of the way God designed people, and the natural rhythm God inbuilt into the world. It is part of how we balance the demands and stresses of life, ensuring that our health remains good and our energy topped up. We are renewed through rest, and this is particularly important at times when we are very busy. Times of rest and relaxation that we plan into our week, far from being time wasted or poorly used, may well be the most important things we do all week.

So what *is* relaxation?

The key to understanding relaxation is to look at what we mean by the term – only then can we understand just why it is so important. For a lot of people talking about relaxation conjures up an image of a room filled with lycra-clad people, chanting with their eyes closed. Relaxation classes and exercises are one way of relaxing – but they are not what relaxation is all about – and the risk is that what they do is make you associate relaxation with something quite difficult, out of your ordinary life, perhaps even a bit weird if you are not the kind of person who would go to those kinds of classes anyway.

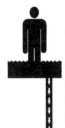

Relaxation is all about finding things to do that offer your body *and mind* the chance to wind down. If you think about that image of yourself standing in a pool where the water level represents your level of stress,[1] relaxation is a bit like pulling the plug out so the water level can drop. Relaxation offers our brain and bodies the chance to 'switch off' – or at least wind down somewhat – after a period of high demand. It counteracts the risk of our stress levels beginning to become chronically raised, and keeps us healthy, energised and ready to go.

Relaxation therefore can be *physical relaxing* – in that it helps our bodies to turn down the physiological components of stress – and/or *cognitively relaxing* – allowing our brains to switch off. Some activities can score high on both. It's good to be aware what activities might be relaxing in which ways – and to realise that these vary between people. For example, for me, taking a nice hot bath can be relaxing in both ways. The warmth of the water is very physically relaxing, and aids muscle relaxation as well as slowing my cardiovascular system and reducing my blood pressure. But the peace and quiet of the room also allows my racing brain the chance to slow down, and shutting the door momentarily on the rest of the world creates an oasis of headspace for me. However, some people find that in the same circumstances their brain – given nothing at all to distract and occupy it – would start to run wild, and obsessive or intrusive thoughts or worries might well become a problem. For this to be a cognitively relaxing experience, they'd need to add something to occupy their brain without it being too taxing. The radio, for example, or a book or magazine to read. It is important that we are self-aware and honest enough to experiment with relaxing activities, and to learn for ourselves which are successful in which ways.

---

1   See Chapter 2 – 'All about *stress*'.

One thing to be aware of is the risk of falling into a trap that I have found to be all too common amongst people I have worked with for stress–related problems. Very often people who are very driven and productive choose things to do in their non-work time which are equally driven and productive! So, they go out running, but unsatisfied with that on its own, train for a marathon, or triathlon. They go to take a bath but take with them their latest management textbook or report they need to read for work. While on the surface they are taking time out, the reality is that they are offering their brains little or no time to relax. Another common 'false friend' along these lines is playing on games consoles. These may be great fun and a very easy way to eat away some leisure time, but with the fast paced, often tense and complex gameplay, they are not very relaxing. In fact they may put your brain in particular even more on alert! There's nothing wrong with playing them, but we need to realise that they are not really cognitively relaxing – and if they are dramatic and tense enough they may even trigger our stress response!

Learning to relax

What is really important to remember is that relaxation, just like anything else, is a skill. It takes time to get good at it, and to get to know yourself and what works best for you. Make a start by planning regular slots into your week for relaxation. Ideally you would make space for it every day (before bed time is a good as it will also help you wind down for sleep), but perhaps start by aiming for 3 – 4 times a week. You can vary when and how you plan these slots – see what works best. But remember the order of the rhythm – work comes first! Most of your relaxation time will follow on from work – in your lunch hour maybe, or after work, in evenings and at the weekend.

Once you have planned some slots into your week ahead, it is time to think about some things to try out. Brainstorm a list of ideas – things that you *might* find relaxing. You won't know until after you have tried how well they work so be creative and think of as many and as varied ideas as you can. Think of things that are physically relaxing, and things that are more cognitively relaxing. Remember that some things might energise you at first, but have a long term relaxing impact – exercise for example. Remember also that you might be able to combine some of these ideas. So, read your book in the bath, or go for a long walk with a friend and catch up at the same time!

Here are a few thoughts/ideas to get you started.

Relaxation ideas:

Things that are physically relaxing	Take a hot bath; go and have a massage; burn an aromatherapy candle while reading; relaxation exercises.
Exercise	Go running/swimming/for a bike ride; play sport with a friend or join a sports team; go to exercise class.
Things that distract you from your worries/occupy your mind	Reading a good (non-work) book, watching a film/going to the cinema; watching TV.
Creative time	Sewing/knitting/embroidery, etc.; learning/practising an instrument; painting; woodwork, etc.
Seeking social support	Meeting up with friends; catching up over a coffee/beer; calling someone on the phone.
Restoring order (N.B. not everyone finds these things relaxing!)	Tidying up a drawer/cupboard; doing the ironing; organising a shelf, etc.

Each time you have a relaxation 'slot' in your week, make a point of trying out one of these ideas. Note that some will take longer than others. So you might not be able to go on a 10 mile bike ride in your lunch hour, but you might be able to go and grab 20 minutes reading quietly on a bench in a park near where you work. Each time you try something, ask yourself how relaxing you found it. Mark it on a scale of 1 to 10, where 10 is really relaxing and 1 is not relaxing at all. Give each idea more than one chance – sometimes things just go wrong – and see how you get on. Soon you will start to get an idea of the simple basic relaxation things you can plan into your week. Bit by bit it will become more natural and less something you have to plan in. But beware – when you get really busy and stressed, that's when you may have to revert to deliberately scheduling or planning these slots in!

What about relaxation classes/techniques?

So, what about those classes or techniques that claim to teach you how to relax? These can be a fantastic thing to build into your relaxation routines throughout the week. But they can't be your *only* source of relaxation. Do include them as part of the things you try, but be aware that as classes, these are techniques that you *learn*. At first you may find them much more difficult, even frustrating, and you may find they are not relaxing at all! But as you get better – and as you get more used to switching off and relaxing because of the other things you have been trying, you will find that they get more helpful.

Some relaxation techniques offer a CD/video/app that you can use at home. These can be really helpful because you can use them if no one else is around. They can be especially helpful in calming anxious thoughts or helping you wind down at the end of the day or if you cannot sleep. Again, try a few out (most libraries have a good selection that you can borrow) and see what works for you.[2]

So about that Sabbath …

And finally, a word about the Sabbath rhythm. We've talked about building rest and relaxation into your life but we haven't specifically mentioned that big challenge – taking a *whole day off* each week. Listen: I know how hard it is. I have a family, a house to keep (vaguely) tidy, people to feed, homework to supervise, various freelance jobs … It would be hard to fit that stuff into eight days, never mind six! But I know how important that rhythm is, so I always try to have one day a week where the work at least is off the menu. That means the laptop goes off, emails are not checked (no, not even on my phone!) and I don't cheat and do research. I use the time for my family and to spend extra time with God – read a bit more of whatever Bible study book I am working through at the time, perhaps listen to a sermon podcast while doing some baking – things that I know are restful and feed my body spirit and soul. I'll be honest: it doesn't work every week. But it is my aim, because I know that it is God's best for me – God's ideal. I also find that imposing that structure on my week forces me to be less sloppy with things the rest of the time: if I know I can't work on that day, I focus more on the other days; perhaps do a bit more writing and less reading of Twitter or that day's news!

Struggling to see how you could plan a regular 'Sabbath' into your week? First of all, remember it doesn't *have* to be Sunday. If you work with the church, or even if you just volunteer, it is highly likely that day will not be all that restful. You might even have to split your Sabbath and maybe have two afternoon

---

2 To get you started, there's a simple relaxation exercise suggested in Appendix 2.

Sabbaths over each weekend, or make sure you take Saturday am and Sunday pm off. Those who do shift work may find it is a different day each week.

If you think you just can't get everything work-wise done in six days, think about keeping a diary for a couple of weeks of how you spend each hour of each day. This may feel like a chore, but it is very interesting and often revealing about how you spend your time. You'll find more on how to do this in the 'over to you' section next. This will reveal exactly what is going on in your week: Are there periods of time you don't use as efficiently as you might? Are there things you do that take longer than they should, or things that intrude upon your work time? Are there things you would need to do in order to protect 'down' time – turn off your phone, for example? It may require you to organise your whole week better, but if you are able to plan so that most of the time you get a clear day off, you and those around you will benefit. Remember, that day could be the most important day of your week!

Most of all, as you think about the Sabbath rhythm, and about rest, remember this – this stuff and these rules aren't there to **stress** you out or **catch** you out – they are there to **help** you out. Don't beat yourself up if it doesn't work out one week. Don't do it because you feel guilty if you don't. Do it because you know God wants the best for you – and because you want to give your best to God.

Over to you ...

Do you keep a regular 'Sabbath day'? (Be honest!) If not, what stops you?

How would *you* define 'relaxation'?

Do you find it easy to relax? Are there particular times/situations when you find it harder?

Do you plan regular activities or slots into your schedule that are just for relaxation? If so, how often?

How often do you think you should be taking time out to relax?

What sorts of things do people do to relax? Think of as many examples as you can!

Do you need to make a decision to plan more relaxation times into your week? If so, try to think of some practical times/slots where you might be able to plan something.

10

Wise building and *emotional* gardening

Relaxation is the best way to counteract and manage stress – but of course what is much more effective is if we can succeed in moderating how we respond to the challenges life throws us and *reduce* the stress we experience. Throughout the book we've been aware that some people may be more prone to stress than others. If this is you, how can you prepare yourself and ready yourself in such a way as to minimise your stress response?

In Matthew 7, Jesus tells one of my favourite parables: it's the story of two men, each building a house. The wise man built his house on a rock. It must have taken a lot of time, digging those foundations into the stone. Probably weeks went by and he had nothing to show for it but a slowly growing hole in the rock. But he got there in the end and finished his house. The other man built on sand. He must have felt he was laughing when he started. His foundations were much easier, so I imagine the house would have gone up faster. Probably he was sitting on his front porch with a cold drink in his hand watching his neighbour still bashing away at the hard, unyielding rock.

But the good weather didn't last. Both men were hit by storms. And here's the difference: the man with his house on the rock weathered the storms. His house (and he) survived.

At the end, when the water subsided and the wind fell back to normal he was still standing. The man who had built on the sand however, lost everything. (Matthew 7:24-29).

What does this have to do with how we handle stress?

Stormy times

For years I read this story, and tucked it away into my head, without really thinking about what it meant. I became increasingly cross and frustrated every time we hit stresses, dramas and the usual crazy and rough times that pretty much every family encounters. I felt like my faith, my living for and serving God, should protect me from such times. I felt like I should be sheltered, somehow, from stress, sailing my little boat across strangely calm seas, even when other people were hitting storms.

I was stupid! This story states one truth more clearly than any other. It doesn't matter who we are or what we build our lives upon - *storms will come*. There will be times in your life where it throws at you things you never expected to be part of your life story - things that make you shout, things that make you cry, things that make you wonder if you can get through another day. I'm not being negative, I am just being realistic. You can do everything right and still sail into a storm. The difference is what happens afterwards.

Have you ever tried to build a house of cards? I have, several times, triggered mainly by a love of Agatha Christie's Hercule Poirot, who builds them in order to help calm and focus his mind. (They don't really calm my mind, probably because they keep on falling down!) Now read how *The Message* translates Jesus' interpretation of his parable: 'If you just use my words in Bible studies and don't work them into your life, you are like a stupid carpenter who built his house on the sandy beach. When a storm rolled in and the waves came up, it *collapsed like a house of cards*' (Matthew 7:26-27, italics mine).

This parable is a wonderful message about something incredibly important – it is about *what we build our lives upon*. Consider Moses' parting words to the Israelites about the laws and commandments God had given them: 'They are not just idle words for you – they are your life' (Deuteronomy 32:47, NIV). This parable offers the same advice about how to respond to Jesus' teachings and wisdom. They are not just to be viewed as clever sayings, wise proverbs or neat metaphors. They are solid rock on which we can build our lives so that when the pressure is on, it doesn't collapse like a house of cards. This isn't the easiest way to build your life, but it is the most stable, and the most resistant to storms.

Notice also that the account of Jesus' telling of this parable begins with that word again: 'therefore'. Before he tells the story, Jesus explains *why* he tells it. Directly before this parable Jesus is teaching all about the difference between true disciples and those who may say everything right, but actually are not entirely genuine. Rather soberingly, Jesus tells those listening, 'wide is the gate and broad is the road that leads to destruction, and many enter through it. But small is the gate and narrow the road that leads to life, and only a few find it' (Matthew 7:13-14, NIV).

Taking time to think about what you build your life upon is not always easy, and it takes time. Most people never stop to think about such things. It also takes considerable effort to resist the messages that our culture throws at us about other things which are important. But this parable advises us to make the effort. We need to be sure that we have built on the one dependable foundation – on God. If right now you are having to take some time out to think about your life and the way you think, act and react, if stress has pulled you up on some emotional shortcomings – be encouraged. Taking this time to put in deep foundations is a great thing to do. It does not mean that you are weak, but it will make you stronger.

What is your life built upon?

In essence, what this parable is about psychologists would call *resilience*. It is that factor which makes us able to stand the storms of life, and come through them still standing. In stress terms it is what makes some people able to manage stressful times well, while others seem to struggle with relatively low levels of stress.

In Chapter 3[1] we looked at some of the differences in the way people think, experience and react to the world - contrasts in the rules or goals accordingly to which some people live. If you look at what underlies these goals, why they are so important to you, that reveals the things which mean the most to you - the things upon which you build your life. For example, consider the person who lives by a rule that says 'I must never make a mistake'. At the root of this rule lies a basic belief about the importance of being (or at least appearing) perfect. This is a value that person is living by. They are building their life upon a foundation which requires them to be perfect - something that by definition they will not manage to maintain. Is it any wonder that such a person is at higher risk of stress?

The temptation to build our lives on such flimsy foundations is all around us. They may feel secure and familiar - but when we are under pressure they cannot take the strain and quickly start to crumble. Watch any ad-break and you can see examples of things upon which our culture encourages us to build our lives. Success, money, our appearance, possessions - these are the things we are sold promising that they will bring us happiness. But they don't, and their weakness will be particularly revealed in times of stress. In fact a recent study found that only one thing reliably predicted happiness in adult life - not money, not possessions, not a big house, not having a top job or a fast car. It was emotional health. Learning to build your life on good strong foundations helps you be resilient, enables you to build

---

1 'Are you a stresshead?!'

and maintain good emotional health and to survive whatever storms you face.

The secret to being happy

In all of this, I want to turn once again to Paul. As we know he was a man who was very driven – and he also comes across as a bit of a perfectionist. Listen to the way he talks about his own frustrations with himself: 'I do not understand what I do. For what I want to do I do not do, but what I hate I do … I have the desire to do what is good, but I cannot carry it out. For I do not do the good I want to do, but the evil I do not want to do – this I keep on doing' (Romans 7:15, 18, 19, NIV). Paul certainly set himself high standards and you can hear his frustration at not being able to live up to them. But he seems to have grasped something significant in the way he manages these frustrations – something from which we can learn a great deal in our study of how to manage stress.

Paul writes an incredible chapter in Philippians 4, where he talks clearly about what he now builds his life upon. He finishes with these words: 'I'm glad in God, far happier than you would ever guess … Actually, I don't have a sense of needing anything personally. I've learned by now to be quite content whatever my circumstances. I'm just as happy with little as with much, with much as with little. *I've found the recipe for being happy* whether full or hungry, hands full or hands empty. Whatever I have, wherever I am, I can make it through anything in the One who makes me who I am' (Philippians 4:10-14, *The Message,* italics mine).

What Paul is describing is the essence of resilience – whatever life throws at him he knows he can get through it. And why? He has built his life on something so solid he can be certain it will carry him through any storm. He has found the recipe for being happy. And what is it? 'I can make it through anything in the One who makes me who I am.' The NIV puts this perhaps more succinctly: 'I can do all this through him who gives me strength.' Paul's recipe for being happy is the same one that Jesus points us towards in the parable of the wise builder: he has built his whole life on the rock – on God.

How do you build your life on God?

In order to understand a bit more about the journey Paul has been on, we can look back through the same letter. After all we know a little of Paul's life story. We know that before he had an experience of God, Paul was a very important man, a high up Roman involved in persecuting Christians. But that changed dramatically after he realised the truth about God. His move into ministry changed everything. He tells the Philippians '...all the things I once thought were so important are gone from my life' (Phil 3:8, *The Message*). Paul has had an experience of losing everything he used to build his life upon. He lists some of the things he had going for him before he came to know Christ: 'You know my pedigree: a legitimate birth, circumcised on the eighth day; an Israelite from the elite tribe of Benjamin; a strict and devout adherent to God's law; a fiery defender of the purity of my religion, even to the point of persecuting the church; a meticulous observer of everything set down in God's law Book' (Phil. 3:4-6). Paul used to get his value, his self-worth and his status from his background, his heritage, but now he has had a revelation about what is really important. He says, 'The very credentials these people are waving around as something special, I'm tearing up and throwing out with the trash – along with everything else I used to take credit for' (vv. 7-8, *The Message*).

Paul has had an incredible experience of God – one that started on the day he heard from God on the road to Damascus, but it didn't end there. It is a journey that he has travelled as he has journeyed in real life, travelling and telling people about God. He has found that the things he believed were important actually are not – and this has blown his mind.

Whilst answering challenges from some of the Jews, Jesus spoke about the kind of change Paul had experienced. He was talking to the Jews who had believed what he had said, and he gave them this advice: 'If you hold to my teaching, you are really my disciples. Then you will know the truth, and the truth will set you free' (John 8:31-32). It is a very well-known verse. But what does it mean by 'knowing' the truth – does it mean that if you learn if by heart it will free you? No, what Jesus says is more than that. He tells them to 'hold on' to his teaching. This is more than just head knowledge – it is building your life on the things Jesus has said. *The Message* translation puts it like this: 'If you stick with this, living out what I tell you, you are my disciples for sure. Then you will *experience for yourselves* the truth, and the truth will free you' (John 8:31-32, italics mine). It is more than knowledge of God and his teaching that brings us to freedom. It is an experience of those truths for ourselves.

This is certainly what has happened to Paul. Carrying on in his letter, his enthusiasm bubbles over. 'I consider everything a loss because of the surpassing worth of knowing Christ Jesus my Lord, for whose sake I have lost all things. I consider them garbage, that I may gain Christ and be found in him, not having a righteousness of my own that comes from the law, but that which is through faith in Christ' (Phil. 4:8-9, NIV). Paul is saying that not only does he now realise that he doesn't want to build his life on those things he once thought important, but he realises now just how unimportant they are. The NIV translates the word he uses as 'garbage' but the actual word is quite a bit stronger than that! Paul's experience of God has totally transformed his perspective on what matters.

So how do we make this same change in ourselves? At the heart it is about an experience of God – something we pray for and journey with throughout our lives. But there is also an element of choice about what we decide to build our life on. For many of us the goals that we live by, and the values that underlie them are things of which we have little awareness. If we are not aware, we act fairly automatically. But once we become aware, everything changes – then we become able to make a choice about how we live, and we can choose to change the things we think are important. We can choose to change what we build our life upon.

Emotional gardening

One approach which helps you to become aware of the way you are living, and the source of your thought patterns is cognitive behavioural therapy (CBT). As we've already explored, CBT looks at the influence that your thinking has on your emotions, and how thoughts can modify your experience of whatever is going on around you. It also helps you to identify the values which underlie your thinking and play a role in triggering emotions as well as helping you manage your emotions better by identifying certain unhelpful styles of thinking, which have been demonstrated to be linked to a higher risk of emotional problems. It then encourages you to challenge those thoughts and gradually reduce their frequency. I like to call CBT emotional gardening – it is about pruning some of our thought patterns and perhaps weeding out the worst offenders: thoughts which are not realistic or rational, and which trigger a lot of negative and difficult emotion.

Interested in these 'unhelpful' thinking styles? Here are just a few which CBT aims to identify:

Having a negative bias. This thinking style is what you might call instinctive pessimism! It assumes the worst probably will happen and focuses on it. So, you probably will catch that cold over your holiday, the train probably will be late and it'll be your bag that gets lost at the airport. We might chuckle at this pattern, but thinking this way generates a lot more emotion and can be associated with high levels of worry. If you consider how few of your worries actually come true, you can see that thinking like this leads you to experience a lot of unnecessary stress.

'All or nothing' thinking. This is quite a common thinking style, and is particularly associated with perfectionism. Here things are either one thing (black) or the other (white). There is no grey. Commonly associated with harsh judgements about oneself (e.g. 'I totally messed that presentation up' when in reality there was only one small error), it often requires complete perfection, or categorises things a 'failure'. All or nothing thinking can be seen in other contexts however, for example in eating ('I've had one spoonful of the ice cream, I may as well eat the whole tub').

I feel therefore I am. We've covered this way of thinking before – mistaking emotions for 'fact' when in reality they are just warnings that something *might* be true. So, I feel guilty so I am guilty; I feel worried therefore that thing I am dreading almost definitely *will* happen…

Catastrophising. This rather wonderful term describes what happens when our thinking becomes carried away by anxiety, resulting in predictions of disaster which then trigger further anxiety. It involves great leaps between what has happened now forwards in time, in each case assuming the worst. Irrational though those leaps are, catastrophising makes it much harder to think rationally, so our reaction is as though the endpoint 'worst case scenario' has actually occurred or is unavoidable. So it might start 'I am going to be late for that meeting', then jump to 'I am going to look a total mess when I get there because I've had to run all the way … People will think I am a total mad person … They will all be wondering why I got the job … If I don't say something really clever they will probably complain about me … I am going to lose the job … I will never get another job … We will not be able to pay the mortgage … We will lose the house' … And so on!

These thinking styles are a bit like having your head full of kindling – they are what catch when the flame of emotion lights up, and they fuel those emotional bonfires which can rage in our heads. The more we can eradicate them, the more in control we will feel, and the better managed our response to stress will be.

Be transformed …

CBT is a secular therapy, but it lies very much in line with biblical teaching. As we explored in Chapter 3,[2] Paul's advice is to 'be transformed by the renewing of your mind' (Romans 12:2, NIV). Understanding your thinking better enables you to examine honestly what you are building your life upon, so that you can decide if you need to make some changes. Paul himself has experienced the difference a change in perspective can make – from a secular set of values to following God's values. *The Message* translation of Romans 12:2 gives the following great advice: 'Don't become so well-adjusted to your culture that you fit into it *without even thinking*. Instead, fix your attention on God. You'll be changed from the inside out' (italics mine).' We need to learn to be better aware of our thoughts, and the values and goals that underlie them – and then be prepared to challenge them. We need to be continually making the conscious decision to base our lives on God, and not on other things. It isn't easy! But each time we succeed, we shore up our foundations so that we weather the next storm better.

---

2 'Are you a stresshead?!'.

Over to you ...

Can you remember times in your life where you hit emotional storms?

How's the weather for you now?! Are there things life is throwing at you right now that might be contributing towards your stress? In the 1960s two psychologists called Thomas Holmes and Richard Rahe came up with a list of life events, giving each a score which related to how stressful it is. Here are just a few (and their scores). They're not all negative events but they do all involve adjustment – and therefore stress!

Tick any which you have experienced in the last 6 months.

Death of a spouse	100	
Death of a close family member	63	
Death of a close friend	37	
Divorce	73	
Marital separation	65	
Marriage	50	
Personal illness/injury	53	
Retirement	45	
Pregnancy	40	
Change in job/work	36	
Change in living conditions	25	
Christmas	12	
A holiday	13	

How's your score? The original study suggested the higher your score the greater the chance of illness because of stress. This list only has a few examples of the kinds of stressful life event life can throw at you. Is there anything else you have experienced recently which has triggered a lot of stress?

Paul lists some of the things he used to build his life on - including his background, some of the life milestones he had experienced, his family history, his faith and his views/passions. What things do you feel the pull/temptation to build your life on?

Did you identify with any of the unhelpful thinking styles this chapter describes? How do you think they affect you, and your stress levels?

11

Careful caring

Back in Part 1, we looked at certain characteristics that can lead to a higher stress load and identified that some people - though they are drawn to caring - experience very high levels of stress from it.

If this is you, what should you do? What should our response to this be, as caring people? Should we avoid acting on our instinct to care? Should we try to care less? No, of course not! But it is no good to the people we care for if we burn out within a few years of starting. We must learn to care wisely, and accept that to do so may sometimes mean challenging our instincts.

So how exactly do you go about caring carefully?

Know yourself

In caring for other people we are understandably focused on *their* needs, emotions and situations. But actually it is crucial that we know ourselves even better before we start to support other people. That's not to say that we need to be in some kind of 'ideal' state before we care for others. But we do need to be wise according to our own situation in what we do or do not offer.

The most important thing for us to be aware of is *why* we are drawn to caring in the first place. We are all called to care for others, and to have compassion on those in need. Prov. 21:13

puts it rather bluntly: 'If you won't help the poor, don't expect to be heard when you cry out for help' (CEV). But there can be many motives behind our caring. Some people care because they fear what might happen if they don't: they do so out of a perceived obligation rather than out of compassion. Others, often those who have grown up in a role where they had to be carers for others, live according to a rule or value that they themselves only have value if they are caring for others. And for some, their own experience of their empathetic pain when they see others going through hard times is so powerful, they almost *have* to try to do something about it.

If any of these apply, I'm not saying that means that you shouldn't do any caring. But it is vital that we are on our guard for what our own potential 'Achilles heel' might be in our caring – that is, if we were going to come unstuck what would it be that pushed us over the edge? Might we be at risk of caring for others so much that we forget to care about ourselves? It is for this reason that many professional 'caring' courses require individuals to go through a course of self-analysis before they start caring for others. It is telling that academic examples of teaching 'compassion training' report that the skill most people find hardest is learning to have compassion *on themselves*. Caring cannot be a case of 'those who can't do – teach' – caring for others must start with caring for and understanding ourselves.

Compassion starts at home

Given that compassion training asks us first to develop better compassion skills for ourselves before trying to offer the same to others, how might we go about this? I have already said we need to be self-aware if we are to care for others. Self-compassion is an important part of self-awareness, and it is surprisingly rare. Self-compassion skills such as being self-nurturing, self-comforting and protecting ourselves appropriately from situations, people or pressures that could be harmful to us emotionally or physically are not about turning ourselves into 'islands', people who do not need anyone else. We were designed at a basic level to need other people, and caring for each other is a vital part of God's design for people. Self-compassion is about becoming more resilient, more able to do more for ourselves. Self-compassion skills build confidence, enable us to be more independent and ultimately make us better carers. It could include things like monitoring your work/life balance and making sure you do get enough down time, how you respond when you are unwell or in need, and how you look after yourself when things are tough. Self-compassion skills are highly significant in the fight against burnout because they make sure you monitor your own state, and also prioritise your own needs just as much as you prioritise those of others. We must not forget ourselves in our rush to care for other people.

Put the most important people first

We need to remember that the reason all of this is so important isn't just about us. Careful caring is also about making sure that the people we care most about do not get left out - our families. I have lost count of the number of people I have treated who grew up in a very caring household - often a Christian household - but felt that no one cared about them very much at all. It isn't easy to do but we must ensure that those closest to us receive a message loud and clear which says that they are the most important to us, that there is no doubt we will always put them first.

It is probably in this area that being 'careful' can have the greatest impact. If we care instinctively, rushing to wherever there is need we may well find that we end up short- changing the people who wait for us at home. Does your family only ever get the 'dregs' of your energy when other people have run you dry? There will always be a need that we could feel we had to attend to. We must put in place careful, thought-out strategies to ensure that we get the balance right.

Keep clear boundaries

All this leads me to think about boundaries. You may have heard talk of 'boundaries' before. But what are they, and what does that mean for those of us who care not as professionals, but as members or leaders of churches?

Boundaries describe the limits of the kind of care you offer a person. They may surround practical things like when and for how long you meet, or when and how someone will be able to contact you. They may also make clear how important factors like confidentiality will work within this relationship, i.e. when, why and how you might need to share things they discuss with you with someone else, for example your senior pastor/minister. However boundaries also have another important role: they explain and make clear how this relationship will work. Boundaries, whether stated explicitly, or just maintained implicitly (i.e. without referring to them), clarify the nature of the relationship.

Let me explain that last one in a bit more detail. When we form friendships, we all automatically and gradually start to offer indications of the boundaries of that friendship. Therefore when I met a woman at a coffee morning last week, I found out she came from a town very close to mine, and got chatting with her; before we parted company I asked if I could take her number. That immediately gives her an important piece of information about my take on the friendship - I would like to at some point take it beyond this first meeting by contacting her. And when I asked for her number I also said 'You should come over for coffee sometime', making it clear what kind of contact I would be making. Throughout friendships we give this kind of information, whether consciously and deliberately ('Do call me if I can help with anything'), or through the way we act (for example by letting someone know we are generally in on Monday mornings if they ever want to drop by for coffee).

In therapeutic settings (e.g. counselling), the nature of the relationship is *not* friendship. Professional boundaries therefore help both parties understand this, as well as clarifying practical details of how the relationship will work. Setting clear boundaries therefore includes explaining that it is not a friendship, and helping the client understand something of what it actually is. This is doubly important in situations where the boundaries are much more confused and there may be considerable questions over what the relationship is – for example, if you are caring for someone who is in your church congregation, it is really important that you both know where you stand – and as the less vulnerable person in the relationship it may well fall to you to make sure this is clear.

Why are boundaries important?

The most important thing about boundaries is that they set up and manage the expectations that both parties have of the relationship. In a friendship scenario this is managed between the two of you and any awkwardness (maybe we've all had those moments when someone clearly wants to be a closer friend than perhaps you had in mind!) is managed one way or another. However in a therapeutic relationship we recognise that the people we support are very vulnerable. They may struggle with issues like trust, and may have been let down or rejected many times before. In addition to this we are asking them to share themselves with us – potentially to make themselves more vulnerable. Good boundaries make the relationship a safe and predictable place where they can do this. They ensure that an individual isn't expecting something that you may be unable to give – that they do not, for example, think that they can contact you any time of any day and you will always be able to talk to them or get back to them straight away. Good boundaries protect people who may be very at risk of what they perceive to be rejection by making clear what our limits are.

As well as this, boundaries have further benefits for the people we support. In counselling or therapy, the process can be very painful, raising or examining very difficult emotions or experiences from past or present lives. Good boundaries enable someone to keep their time in therapy very clearly separated from the rest of their life. This is not a friend who they may run into in the supermarket, and have to say hello to. This is a safe space separate from the rest of their life where they can step out of their life and examine the most difficult parts of it. Then at the end of each session they can put those things away again until the next time they enter that space. These kind of clear boundaries are particularly essential when the things someone needs to work through are very traumatic or emotionally triggering.

A third important aspect to clear boundaries is to protect expectations that might otherwise be perceived by the person we are supporting. People in distress are often at their limit in what they can do and take on. A supportive relationship shouldn't expect anything of them; it is very rightly one way, unlike a friendship which asks for more balance. Your counsellor/doctor/ psychologist is not a friend – this is not someone whose birthday you need to remember! The nature of this boundary takes the pressure off the person you are supporting and allows them to relax into a relationship which is, uniquely, totally one way, to care for and be interested in them alone.

A final, often overlooked aspect of boundaries, however, is not for the person we are supporting – it is for *us*! Boundaries protect *us* – and ultimately make sure we are able to keep on caring, and offering the best kind of support. Boundaries keep us sane; they make sure we have space in our lives where we are not disturbed by work calls or people in need. They protect our families, ensuring we have a safe space which isn't invaded by our work, and they help us keep balance, making sure we recharge our batteries and avoid the all too present risk of burnout and compassion fatigue. Even Jesus sometimes walked away from need because he and/or the disciples needed to eat (Mark 6:31), pray (e.g. Luke 5:16, 6:12), rest (Luke 8:23) or just process their own emotions (Matthew 14:13). Do not make the mistake of thinking you will not have the same limits.

Avoid manipulation

A difficult but very important subject to consider here is the sometimes unhelpfully named one of 'manipulation.' I don't really like this term because it suggests that the person in question is fully aware of what is going on, perhaps even deliberately manipulating the situation, and in my experience although manipulation is quite a common issue to deal with in (for example) pastoral care, that is almost never the case. Manipulation describes what happens when someone is caught in a very difficult place, often struggling with self-esteem and having been a victim of abuse or trauma in their past. This, and a lifetime of being 'needy' have taught them that the only reason people care for them is because of their needs. This can lead them – particularly when times are hard – to exhibit very powerful, what I call 'provocative' emotions, which can feel 'designed' to force someone to respond, whether that is just by paying attention to them, or to do something specific – come round to see them, for example. Alternatively, manipulative behaviour can be about setting you up to fail, when the person you are caring for is convinced they are not worth your attention and wants to prove that you 'do not really care'. They may engineer situations where you do not meet their needs (e.g. not realising they are upset, not responding to calls, etc.) in order to 'prove' to themselves that they are right.

Being on the receiving end of manipulative behaviour is extremely stressful. You may feel like you are suddenly an actor in a drama you never intended to perform in, suddenly responsible for someone's welfare in a way you never expected. You may find it triggers a very strong emotional – and stress – reaction in you. Calls for help may well come in at times that are very difficult, evenings and weekends for example, and you may feel that you cannot refuse to respond. You may find yourself 'set up' to fail, and accused of not caring. Manipulative behaviour can very quickly burn out well-meaning people, who give and give until they can give no more. Sadly when they then have to stop, this is perceived as a rejection, making things even worse for the vulnerable person.

Boundaries are absolutely key in avoiding manipulation. They clearly and carefully set the expectation from the start, and make sure both parties know what to expect. The difficult thing is that people who can be manipulative often 'push' the boundaries. So they might say things like 'I know I am not supposed to call you at the weekend, but …'. We need to appreciate that this is not done deliberately – it's because the strength of their emotions and the panic and anxiety that people might reject them lead them to push the limits and ask for help at different times. They may feel that they cannot cope on their own, so at times when they know your help is not available this might feel more powerful and lead them to get in touch.

However tempting it may be, do not give in! Maintaining the boundary helps them as well as you – helping them gain confidence that they can manage until your next time together, and developing skills which are good emotional coping strategies, like ways of 'holding' what they are feeling, until they are able to share it with someone. Think about using deliberate tools for this – a diary often works well. They write in the diary when they are feeling desperate and then bring it to times they meet with you – this helps them learn to delay sharing what they feel but also helps get their emotions 'out of their head' in the moment.

Responding healthily to manipulation may feel cruel, like you are abandoning people when they are most in need. It may even lead to other people (usually less well-boundaried people!) accusing you of being uncaring. But this is central to the number one rule of careful caring: we must never care for people in such a way that leads them to become more dependent on us. If we do, we are helping them *remain unwell,* and that is what would be truly uncaring, because their situations are often desperately sad. We must care in such a way as to help them gain and regain independence, confidence and self-esteem. Then we support them to make positive changes to their life and hopefully to see gradual, but positive change.

What about church leaders/pastoral care?

You may well be thinking that this talk about boundaries is all very well, but you do not offer any 'professional' caring role. You may care 'just' as a friend, member of the church or in your capacity as a home group leader, vicar or pastor. You may well not have an office where people come to see you, and there may well be actual overlaps in your life and that of those you care for – you probably have friends in common, or children who attend the same parties. So how do these boundary practices apply to you? Your role may well mean that your boundaries cannot be as clear – but that makes it extra important that you are aware of them, and deliberate in setting them, and maintaining them. Without clear boundaries you run the risk of heading into very difficult and potentially emotionally draining situations where one person's expectation is very different to what another is able to or willing to offer. Stopping to think about the way you care, and what your boundaries may or should be, is a vital stage in caring wisely.

One important question is whether this 'grey' quality to some of our boundaries means that we shouldn't be offering support to people. Those who come from professionally trained backgrounds may shudder to think of operating within such blurred boundaries. However, I personally believe there is a particular strength to working in these 'grey' areas. We are called to be more than 'professional carers' – we are called to share our lives with people. But this emphatically doesn't mean that we don't need to pay attention to boundaries. In fact it means we have to be even more careful and deliberate about them.

How to set good boundaries for pastoral care

Good boundaries for pastoral care acknowledge the grey areas, but set clear expectations for both sides. Here are some things you should think about:

When and how someone can contact you. Be clear. What phone number? Email or text? What times of day? Also think about being clear about when you will respond. 'Not straight away' is a good answer to this! Make clear you may not always have access to messages, etc., and it may be a few days before you can respond. Also make clear when you have family times/days off, etc., and would ask them to hold on and contact you the next day.

What to do in a crisis. Some people you support will be literally on the edge. For these people it is essential to think about what they do in a crisis and who they call (especially if it isn't able to be you!). Do you have a church office number that is staffed by volunteers? Or a 'crisis phone' held by whoever is on duty that day/evening? If not then make sure they are aware of other 'out of hours' crisis options. If they are in contact with the local mental health team they will have a crisis number if not, make sure they know about other options like the Samaritans http://www.samaritans.org, or premier lifeline http://www.premier.org.uk/life/lifeline.aspx.

What you (and the church) can (and importantly can't) offer. It is really important that we are realistic and recognise our limits. You may want to push the limits in terms of how you care for people but as long as you are human you will never be able to escape them entirely. Be clear about what you can offer

– not treatment or therapy, just support, consistency, the space to talk, and prayer. And if someone pushes your limits – calling out of the blue, say, don't turn them away entirely, but don't be on call 24 hours a day, 7 days a week. Instead plan a time when you can talk to them and give them your full attention – the support they deserve.

When they will see you. We need to be clear about this – when we arrange time specifically for them to talk, think and/ or to pray with them we must be clear. Always cover *where* you will meet. (Some meetings are very well suited to the local coffee shop. Others are not. Check first!) Make clear *when* you will meet – *start and finish times!* You do not want them just to be getting into the flow of things after 45 minutes when you had another appointment booked in! Be clear! Learn how to gently reinforce this – ten minutes before the end of your time warn them. ('We need to finish soon; is there anything else you particularly wanted to talk about today?') And do be wise; 5 minutes before you have to go is not the time to ask a particularly triggering question or to unlock a really painful memory. Remember they have to go back to their lives, so make sure they leave you in an appropriate state for this.

What will happen/how to react when they run into you/encounter you in other circumstances. This is so important in our 'grey' world. I always warn people they will see me in church and we chat about how we will both react. Some prefer to ignore me, which is fine. I warn them that sometimes people assume if they know someone knows me, that they have some kind of issue they are working through, so those who are really private prefer not to be saying hello on Sundays, which is fine by me. More usual though is that we agree to say a brief 'Hi', and leave it at that.

Not with haste …

Careful caring is not about caring less. Instead it is about caring wisely. I love the way a Mumford and Sons song puts it: we need to resolve to '*love with urgency but not with haste*'.[1] Caring is an essential part of our role as God's ambassadors on this earth, and that makes it doubly important that we do it in a measured, appropriate way. Caring wisely ensures that we are able to continue it long term, being more effective carers, and also has a significant role to play in how we manage stress.

---

1 'Not with haste' - from the album *Babel*.

Over to you ...

How involved would you say you are in caring for other people?
Tick any of the following which apply to you:

I am the main carer for 1/more children
I am the main carer for an adult in my family
I am on the pastoral care team
I do a lot of 'un-official' caring in my church/elsewhere

Would you say you are a 'naturally' caring person?

My caring is very
instinctive.   My caring is very
I don't put a lot of   planned
thought into why/   I think a lot about
what I do   what I do and why

Are there particular situations that you find emotionally much
more difficult than others when you are caring for/supporting
someone else?

Do you care for yourself as well as you care for other people (e.g. making sure you get enough sleep/time to rest)?

What would your partner/a close friend say if we asked them the same question about you?

Do you think the people closest to you (family, friends) ever miss out on anything because of your caring for others?

Take some time to think about the boundaries you set around your caring – whether it is as someone in a 'formal' role (e.g. pastoral caring) or more informal. Think about each of these:

How people contact you: What phone numbers/details do you tend to give out? Can people always get in touch with you? Might you need to protect times when they cannot (e.g. family times so you cannot be disturbed)?

How long you spend with people: Whether meetings or phone calls, etc. – are you clear about how much time you have available? Do you set a time you need to finish by and stick to it? Are you ever late for other things because you 'cannot escape' from a caring situation?

Crisis situations: If you needed to, do you know who you would call in a crisis, if someone you were supporting needed help you were unable to give?

What can (and can't) you offer? Are you clear on what the limits are on your caring – practical (e.g. time, other demands on you); emotional (making sure you get time for you as well as them) and physical (making sure you do not end up as exhausted as the person you are supporting). Are there other people who can 'share the load' so that you can get/take breaks when you need to? If not, where could you look for people who might be able to help you care for this person?

Do you think you need to be more proactive (i.e. planned) in your caring, rather than reacting to whatever is thrown at you? Can you think of specific situations/challenges/areas where you might need to do some research/reading/ask advice so you can plan in advance how to handle them?

12

Don't *blow your top!*

If you are stressed out, the chances are that the people around you know about it - mainly due to the increase in one particular group of emotions. Anger, aggression, frustration, irritability - all are inextricably associated with stress. All harness the same 'fight or flight' system, but with one key feature. Whereas anxiety is experienced mainly in terms of the unpleasant physical sensations and experiences it produces, anger and its associated emotions, with the emphasis very much on 'fight', usually cause problems because of *what they lead us to do*.

In research about emotion, one hypothesis about their function is that they set up what is called 'action tendencies'; that is they make us more likely to act in certain ways. This means that when there is a need for us to do something - to deal with a potential situation or outcome that would conflict with a goal or value that is important to us - emotions nudge us towards actions that might change things. Anger makes us much more likely to do things like hit out, shout, act aggressively, challenge and argue. It can be a very powerful emotion, at times explosive and overwhelming. It can lead us to act in ways which we would never normally.

Anger hijack

Emotions are designed to grab our attention. The physiological changes they trigger make us stop what we are doing and draw our attention to what is going on around us. At the same time, our thinking brain is alerted, and begins to analyse the situation. The combination of these things leaves us well placed to make a decision – do we need to act or not? But most people know from experience that anger can quickly wipe out our ability to think clearly. The more prone you are to bursts of anger and frustration – the more you risk experiencing 'emotional hijack'[1] – acting literally without thinking, out of some primitive fighting instinct. Only once you have cooled down will you have the opportunity to think about what you did – and chances are you won't feel great about it.

Type A personality?

One thing you may have heard mentioned in relation to stress and anger/frustration is discussion of what is called 'Type A' personality. This is a personality type characterised by the readiness with which the person becomes angry and irritable. Their approach to life tends to be very conflict based, and they will often manufacture situations where disagreements or discussions are decided in very conflict intense ways. Type A personalities hold some apparent advantages – they are very hard working and focused people who often achieve great things. They can also be confident people who operate well in competitive environments and are not put off by challenges or difficulties they may experience.

Type A/B personality theory ('Type B' people show a much more laid back approach to life) came to prominence in the 1970s when research began to identify significant results

1 See Chapter 3, 'Are you a stresshead?!'

showing an increased risk of coronary heart disease and other heart problems in people who scored as highly 'Type A'. The theory was that their hostile, aggressive model of living placed them at higher risk of chronic stress. Though their personality and emotional make-up meant that they might not experience this as emotionally stressful (indeed some might even thrive off it), the physical consequences of this long term heightened stress level began to become apparent.

Type A/B personality theory, much as others, has its critics. There has been some evidence in its support, but others criticise the early studies which backed up the theory. It might therefore not be that helpful to obsess too much over whether or not you have or demonstrate 'Type A' features. However, in terms of what we know about stress, it may well be useful to consider how much your own levels of anger, frustration and irritation may be adding to your daily stress. We all have triggers – things which drive us *crazy* and make us really mad, but which might bother other people a lot less. What is interesting is to consider whether any of yours might be contributing to your stress problem at the moment, or meaning that you have to manage a lot of anger and frustration – perhaps more than others.

It is also worth considering whether features of your life make you more at risk of stress because unavoidably your days are spent dealing with well-known frustration triggers – particularly if your role means that you are not able to express that frustration. School teachers, for example, are often continually dealing with low-level disruption or managing the various frustrations of their job. Parents spending most of their waking hours trying to negotiate with tantrum-ridden toddlers, commuters dealing with cancelled or delayed trains – these are all stressful situations to be in because of the frustration they generate. And research into 'Type A' personality tells us is that how you manage that frustration might be very important for your health.

What does the Bible say?

The biblical view of anger is very interesting. The first and very important place to start is to recognise that anger, like anxiety, is a healthy and acceptable emotion to experience. It is not sinful or wrong in essence. Christians have become so tied up with the 'meek and mild' stereotype that some believe it is never right to be angry. This, of course, is not true. Jesus was God in a human body, operating with the limitations and experiences of a human brain, but without sin. He experienced a whole host of emotions including anger. However, the Bible does suggest strong caution in how we *react* to our anger. 'In your anger, do not sin' advises Ephesians 4:26 (NIV), carrying on to suggest that we limit the duration of our anger – 'don't let the sun go down while you are still angry'. Psalm 37:8 advises the same caution around anger suggesting that the risk of a bad reaction is so great, we need to learn to control it better: 'Don't be angry or furious. Anger can lead to sin' (CEV) and Proverbs 27:4 shows an awareness of how powerful anger can be: 'An angry person is dangerous …' (CEV).

In addition to this, there is an interesting theme of contrasting the way God experiences anger with our human tendency to respond to it. Frequently, God is described as 'slow to anger' (for example, Psalm 86:15), and we are advised to try to be the same (e.g. in Ecclesiastes 7:9). The letter written by James, full of challenging teaching about how to live a holy life, directly contrasts the way we might tend to respond with anger to this: 'Everyone should be … slow to become angry, because human anger does not produce the righteousness that God desires' (James 1:19-20, NIV). What that means, in essence, is that our human anger very often produces results that have very little to do with things God wants put right. When Jesus became angry and acted on it it was directly related to things that needed changing with his godly perspective. The reality is that our anger and frustration might be directed at things *we* wish were different, but they tend to be on a slightly lower level than true 'righteous anger'.

Overall, the biblical consensus is clear. There are plenty of examples of people who do slip into very sinful actions because of their anger. Anger must be controlled, and measured; only 'Fools give full vent to their rage' (Prov. 29:11, NIV). This is a clear contrast to the kind of 'emotional hijack' anger we've been thinking about. We definitely don't have a freedom to express our anger however or whenever we want to. Proverbs 9:11 comments that, 'Fools vent their anger, but the wise quietly hold it back' (NLT). Appropriate control of anger is part of emotional and spiritual maturity. We must learn to control and moderate our anger so that we can save it for situations where it is truly deserved.

The big problem: Denial doesn't work.

From all this it is easy to see how a lot of people struggle with anger. Particularly if you have experienced situations in your past (or present) which are triggering, quite understandably, a lot of anger, the anxiety about dealing with it in the wrong way leads a lot of Christians to simply try and pretend their anger is not there. The problem is that this doesn't work. The job of anger is to get your attention. If you try to ignore it it will not just go away. Instead, you may well find that it escalates. Anger can then spill over into other areas of your life: because you are fighting not to admit anger about one thing, you become easily irritated by everything else in your life. Or, because you cannot allow yourself to respond to anger, it may be expressed as a more 'acceptable' emotion such as sadness. Finally anger that cannot be released outwardly often turns inward and directed against ourselves. When this happens the true source of the anger becomes lost, so you just feel more and more frustrated with yourself. This can build up into self-hatred, which can in turn trigger things like self-harm – even though the true fault is nothing to do with you.

Because denying anger doesn't work, we need to deal with it in other ways. We must either cut it off at the source, in developing our understanding of what makes us angry, why, and whether there is anything we need to change here, or we must learn how to modify and control our anger, dealing with the physical changes and sensations it produces and developing positive strategies for expressing it healthily and appropriately.

The anger line - where are you?

Like a lot of emotions, we often get caught out by anger because we only notice it when it is too late. Think of your anger level as somewhere on a line from 0-10, where 0 is no anger/frustration and 10 is the most angry you could ever be. Hopefully right now you are fairly low down the line (assuming this book is not annoying you too much!), but think about the last time you were angry or frustrated and ask yourself what number on the line you were then? Think about how that anger felt – what thoughts were going through your mind and how you were reacting. Did you do anything – shout, stamp your foot, anything else? What kind of thoughts were racing through your head? Did you feel in control or out of control?

We all have a point in our anger, where we become at risk of losing control and being hijacked. This generally lies somewhere around the 8/9 point. If you think of your anger rising a bit like lava in a volcano, this is the point where the pressure has built up so much there is a very real risk that it is going to blow. As we get nearer to this point, it becomes harder and harder to do anything to try to manage our anger – and eventually there is a point of no return where 'eruption' is inevitable. If we try to intervene too late, we are doomed to fail. Whatever strategies you want to try in order to deal with your anger, they will work much better if you can start to use them earlier, when your anger is lower down the line.

Another thing that changes when you draw near to the 'point of no return' is the ability to think and analyse things in complex ways. When your brain is under the influence of such high levels of emotion, it simplifies the way it perceives things – including conflicts – into very black and white scenarios. So, while the real reason your teenager is yelling at you is a combination of hormones, his bad day, his frustration at the fact you were right that he should have spent longer over his homework, the bad grade he got, and the fact that you have now asked him to empty the dishwasher, once in the middle of the fight, your mind will simplify it to 'If I had brought him up properly, he would empty the dishwasher. He isn't doing it; therefore I must be a terrible parent.' Similarly your brain will view anyone involved in a conflict as one of two things: either for or against you. It will struggle to see shades of grey. So when your friend tries to explain why your boss is mad with you, it may feel overwhelmingly shocking that he has sided with your boss and devastating to be let down by him. The truth, of course is not quite that dramatic, but in those moments of hotheaded anger we are anything but rational. Watch out for signs that this is happening to you – thinking or speaking in terms of either 0 per cent or 100 per cent, e.g. 'You *never*'/'You *always*', feeling that everyone is against you, setting 'challenges' – 'If they are really on my side they will agree with me now'/'If they really care they will come and see if I am ok.'

All this means that one very useful tool in managing anger is to become better at identifying it sooner and taking action *before* we get to crisis point. Try making a point of pausing regularly throughout your week and noting where on the line you are. Are you more prone to anger at particular times of day? Are there key things that can be relied upon to frustrate you? As you grow in your understanding of your anger and frustration pattern, you can plan ahead, not just in terms of identifying anger earlier, but potentially making modifications to your plans or schedule in order to relieve some typical anger/frustration pressure points.

Once you become aware that your anger is growing, there are four important approaches to anger to consider:

1 - Bail out!

This first option is by far the simplest, and also both the most effective, and the most sensible. Get yourself out of the situation and take a break. If you know something is going to push you over the edge eventually, don't hang around and wait for it to happen. Act – and do so long before you get to that 'blow your top' point. Remember, the longer you leave it the harder it will get to act. Having removed yourself from the triggers of your anger, it will fall naturally, and as it does so, very quickly your ability to think clearly and sensibly will improve leaving you much more able to act in a rational and constructive manner. This is where the concept of time out comes from for toddlers, but it can be equally useful for adults. (I am often tempted to use the 'one minute for every year you have been alive' rule personally and take breaks of well over half an hour!). It doesn't need to be a long break; often even just five minutes works wonders. You don't need to leave the situation permanently, just give yourself a moment of calm. Pop to the loo, make everyone a coffee, take a moment out of a traffic jam to buy a coffee – whatever it takes. You will often find that just removing yourself from the situation for a short time massively improves your ability to handle it well.

2 - Chill out!

This is of course an essential tool in managing any stress-related emotions: relaxation skills. Learning how to relax yourself and dampen down those stress hormones will help you keep a handle on your anger, and may even reduce it once it starts to bubble over. The key is to combine general good practice in terms of making sure you are fitting regular rest and relaxation into your schedule with 'on the spot' techniques you can use in those moments where someone or something is really winding you up.

'On the spot' is where some of the often-suggested approaches to managing anger can be helpful. Many of them offer quick ways of distracting yourself (slowing the speed with which anger is rising), or dealing with some of the physical 'side effects' of anger (e.g. deep breathing). Don't forget how important motivation is here: you may have good intentions in terms of managing your anger but one showdown with that truly challenging colleague and it all goes to pot. Remind yourself of why this is important – think about learning one of the Bible verses that relate to anger, or get yourself a visible reminder of a reason you want to handle anger better – something that reminds you of your children, or a reminder of a time when anger didn't lead you anywhere good. Sometimes any object can help to remind you of your good intentions even if it doesn't have any particular meaning. Some people swear by wearing an elastic band or similar around their wrist which they can ping in moments where they need to 'snap out of it' and control their anger better. Again, be creative and try different things out until you find what works for you.

3 - Figure it out!

Once again, the third and probably most long term effective option is the more involved and complex: learning what fuels your anger, and developing some good strategies for moderating and expressing your anger more healthily. Here keeping a diary can be really useful. Note down each time you have a real episode of problematic anger – perhaps because you know you totally lost it, or because you did something you really regret or because of the impact it had on you in terms of how you feel.

Write down what happened (including anything that had been significant running up to the event), and how you responded to it. Also note any thoughts you remember going through your head. Over time the diary will help you identify patterns and themes in your thinking, but also in what is triggering your anger.

However, where anger is concerned it isn't only isolated incidents we need to consider when looking at what provoked a crisis. Think of anger as a bit like a river which eventually goes over a waterfall. At the crisis end of things it is a roaring torrent, out of control, hard to swim against and almost always wins out in the end. But if you go back upstream, things become calmer – and smaller. In fact while every big river has a source somewhere, usually they grow up to their largest point because many smaller streams flow into them. Anger is much the same, and it is often the combination of different things having an impact which can lead us to going over the edge. Some sources of anger and frustration in your life may be difficult or impossible for you to eradicate. Others however, may be much more within your control. Identify the smaller streams and take action where you can to reduce your overall anger load and you will find yourself much less likely to be provoked.

Once again when trying to understand anger better, it is also worth being aware of how your thought patterns influence your anger, specifically how they might sometimes magnify anger in certain situations. Watch out for specific tendencies that can magnify frustration in particular – for example the 'if only's (e.g. 'If only I had taken the other road we would never have got stuck in this traffic jam'), the 'shoulda coulda's ('I *should* have realised that this would happen'/'I *could* have sent that email yesterday then this would never have happened') and the character assassination strategies, either of your own or someone else's (e.g. 'I am such an idiot for having let this happen'/'She is totally incompetent and is 100 per cent to blame for this'). All of these can be responsible for raising something frustrating into a complete anger crisis.

4 - Let it out!

Having managed your anger in the moment, don't forget how important it is to find healthy and appropriate ways of expressing it later on, giving an outlet to the pent up frustration which may have built up during the day. You need to release the pent up energy that all the frustration and anger have stored up, but it doesn't have to be released in an angry way. Exercise can be one positive way: anything that gets the blood pumping. If it doesn't need too much control that's even better – sports like tennis can be doubly frustrating when you are angry as overhitting the ball means you don't play very well! Think about more forgiving sports like squash, or ones which allow you to 'pound out' energy such as running or cycling. Sports like these also release naturally relaxing hormones which help to counteract a frustrating day or week, and can lift mood if you are struggling with feeling low or depressed. Otherwise be creative about how you can release that frustration: research ideas and suggestions to try and note down which ones are most successful for you.

Finally, don't forget your psychological need for an outlet. You were never designed to face life on your own, and when it is driving you crazy you certainly need other people around you to share the load. Studies show that seeking social support – chatting things over with friends, or even just making contact via text or email can help us to modify and manage difficult emotions. But be careful just what you do when you offload. Instead of giving in to a torrent of frustration about whoever or whatever is bugging you, try to use the time to think about your own view of the situation and see if there are other perspectives or ideas your friend(s) can offer. Be open to the fact that they might not see it as annoying as you do, and use their knowledge of you to help you try to understand why exactly it is having that effect on you.

Keep safe

Anger can be a powerful emotion, and when levels rise up to crisis point, sometimes they can lead us to act in ways which put either ourselves or other people at risk. If you know you are sometimes at that point, if something is pushing you that far, or if you have had thoughts of harming yourself or others, do not hesitate but get help now. When you are that inundated with an emotion like anger your mind cannot think clearly, and situations can feel more complex and more hopeless than they really are. Don't wait and see how things go the next time: you never know when you are going to be overwhelmed. Find someone to talk to about how you are feeling: visit your GP or call one of the helplines recommended in the resources section.

Over to you ...
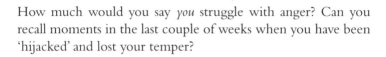

How much would you say *you* struggle with anger? Can you recall moments in the last couple of weeks when you have been 'hijacked' and lost your temper?

How would you have handled things differently had you been able to stay calm?

Are there particular situations/things/people that often make you struggle with keeping your temper?

Do you ever feel guilty about your anger, or that you should hide it?

How often do you feel anger towards yourself?

Here is an anger line:

| 1 | 2 | 3 | 4 | 5 | 6 | 7 | 8 | 9 | 10 |

Where on the line are you RIGHT NOW? What does that feel like? Make some notes below…

Where do you think your own 'point of no return' is – that point at which you lose control? Mark it on the line. What does that feel like – how do you know when you are about to lose it?

Thinking about the 0 – 5 zone on the line. What are some of the warning signs that you are getting angry. What kind of things could you do whilst still in this zone in order to calm down, or stop things getting worse?

Can you think of times when you have been hijacked? If you lived those moments again, how could you do them differently in order to manage your anger – and your actions – better?

13

Why *worry?*

Anger is an emotion which often causes problems in terms of what people *do*. But there is another emotion strongly associated with stress which is much more of a problem in terms of how people *feel*: anxiety/worry.

Wondering what the difference is between anxiety and worry? After all they could be argued as forming part of the same system. To some degree what we're talking about depends on how you use the words, but in general, and in research terms, *worry* is a term used to describe a pattern of thinking, often obsessive or hard to switch off, which fills your mind. This thinking may well fuel *anxiety* – which is usually described as more of an emotional experience, including the physical 'symptoms' of anxiety which we would all recognise. Of course one often feeds another, something research confirms.

Friend *and* foe

Of all our emotions, anxiety is probably the one that we most would like to be rid of. It's ironic therefore that it is probably the one which is most essential. Anxiety arises whenever your brain detects that there is a risk of something happening which is contrary to the goals or values you live by – whether it is your life being threatened, or the chances of you catching the train you're booked on. What determines whether it is useful or not are two things: (1) Whether or not the anxiety triggered is proportional (i.e. is your anxiety system over-reactive, setting off false alarms?) and (2) what your strategies are to deal with the anxiety. Anxiety can be such a powerful experience, and we can experience it so negatively that some of us become what is generally described as *intolerant* of it – that is we would do almost anything in an attempt to be rid of it.

It's understandable that we tend to act to avoid things that make us anxious. But perhaps the most tricky feature of anxiety is that this instinctive reaction actually makes anxiety *worse* rather than better. To understand why you need to think about what is going on at a brain level. Let's say that when you are a child you have a bad experience with a dog. It jumps up at you, or even bites you. In your brain a link is made between the concept of 'dog' and the fact that 'bad things happen'. You might not even need to experience these 'bad things' – if the significant adults in your life react badly every time a dog is around this link can still be made, and reinforced each time they react that way. Eventually, when you meet a dog, that link 'bad things happen' lights up and your brain therefore triggers anxiety.

The next thing you do, understandably, is start to avoid dogs – because you don't want to experience either the anxiety, or the 'worst case scenario' (WCS) that you dread happening again. But the trouble is that this forms another link in our mind which says – in effect – 'The only reason that the WCS didn't happen is that you avoided the dog.' The more you avoid dogs, the stronger this belief becomes. You come to believe that if you ever did come face to face with a dog, the WCS would almost definitely happen; the only reason it hasn't happened so far is because you have been careful.

What I am describing here is the typical formation of one kind of anxiety. Phobias in particular develop this way, but so can other anxieties. Research has shown that this type of emotional reaction to something is incredibly easy to learn, i.e. it becomes fixed in our brains very quickly. We know that avoidance also makes anxiety *grow* very quickly, both in terms of the *degree* of anxiety we experience if we ever are confronted with the thing we are scared of, and of the *level* or *amount* of avoidant behaviour we show. So at first you just try not to stop or have to stand by dogs, but soon you have to cross the road to avoid them, and it isn't long before even seeing them on the other side of the park is a bit scary, and hearing one barking triggers immediate panic.

Anxiety fires

Another form of anxiety disorder is by nature much less specific, and involves a general raised level of anxiety without a specific cause. This heightened state of anxiety can also be called 'free floating' anxiety – where we do not know what is causing it. Free floating anxiety means you exist in a constant state of red alert, never able to totally relax, but never sure what is causing it, and unable to rationalise your way out. Your brain is triggering anxiety *too often* – like an over-sensitive smoke alarm, and on top of that often the sparks of anxiety are then setting fire to great anxiety bonfires as they trigger unhelpful thinking, worrying and what is called 'rumination'. Rumination is what happens when your attention becomes glued to your worries and you find it very hard to shake your thinking onto anything else. Your thinking brain is working overtime – but instead of allowing you to come to a decision over whether you need to take any action, it has become circular, repeating over and over the same thoughts and trapped in a whirlwind of worries. This whirlwind soon fans the flame of anxiety into a blaze.

Fires of anxiety can start much like any other emotional bonfire[1] – but once started they have one special feature. Anxiety blazes act like forest fires – they spread very quickly. As we try to avoid the anxiety trigger, we find we keep needing to 'step up'

---

1 see chapter 3, Are you a stresshead?!

our tactics as other things also start to trigger anxiety. As our fear and dislike of being anxious grows, our general anxiety and stress levels rise, placing us at risk of being 'hypervigilant' (constantly on edge) and experiencing more frequent anxiety triggers as we go about our everyday life. We can quickly end up 'running scared' from anxiety itself. In this way anxiety can come almost from nowhere and very quickly start to cause serious problems.

Who is at risk?

Anxiety problems can hit almost anyone, but some people are statistically at greater risk. A tendency to be anxious or to worry, and certain anxiety related conditions (like obsessive compulsive disorder for example) can run in families, meaning that if a close relative of yours suffers you are statistically at a higher risk of developing it than the general population.

Anxiety problems are also more common in people who are very intelligent and with very active brains – this may be why they are so prone to problems with excessive worry or rumination. Perfectionism is highly associated with anxiety, largely because its high standards leave perfectionists constantly feeling at risk of what they define as 'failure'. In some cases attempts to use perfectionism to deal with problematic anxiety (for example performing checking routines, etc.) can backfire as the anxiety grows, meaning people can become trapped in repeated behaviour (checking more than once, checking even more things, etc.).

Anxiety is also very often strongly linked to stress. Sharing the same physiological system, if you are under sustained stress over a period of time, as your baseline levels of hormones, etc. rise, so does the activity of your anxiety system. This may result in symptoms of anxiety that are greater than you usually experience, or in problematic anxiety in situations where you wouldn't usually feel any. Some people describe suddenly feeling overcome with anxiety or panic and not knowing why.

Panic

One common presentation for stress-related anxiety is for it to first make its presence felt by an 'out of the blue' panic attack. Panic attacks present with what can become dramatic physical symptoms. People experiencing their first can be convinced (as can witnesses) that they are having a heart attack, or that something else is seriously wrong. The symptoms of panic attacks include chest pain, dizziness, numbness or tingling in hands and fingers, nausea and occasionally vomiting or passing out.

A panic attack occurs when the levels of stress or anxiety hormones in your blood get high enough that they start to cause very clear and potentially quite alarming physical symptoms. This may be because of something happening in that moment which suddenly triggers an anxiety 'spike', or it could be because the gradual buildup of stress suddenly means you become aware of a physical symptom. What happens next is that the person experiencing the symptoms of the anxiety/stress becomes aware of them, but misreads them. Instead of identifying that they are due to anxiety, s/he starts to worry that they may be a sign of something else. This triggers further anxiety, which in turn makes the symptoms worse – and very soon a vicious circle results.

One key aspect of panic attacks is the impact they have on your breathing. When we are anxious, our breathing tends to change and become shallower, with more frequent breaths. This mobilises more oxygen should we need to fight or run, but it also means we lose more carbon dioxide than usual. The levels of carbon dioxide in our blood are very important and the drop in these levels itself results in further physical symptoms. These then add to those caused by the anxiety to further convince the person experiencing the panic attack that something really bad is happening.

The treatment of panic attacks is actually fairly simple: once the person is able to calm down, particularly calming their breathing down and returning to a normal rhythm, they should see an improvement in their symptoms. Harder to treat though is the psychological aspect. Many people dread another panic attack, especially if the first was very dramatic. They frequently begin to avoid whatever they perceived to be the trigger. This avoidance increases their anxiety, and particularly if the trigger is hard to avoid, can very quickly mean that the anxiety becomes a big problem.

The good news is that panic attacks can respond quickly to treatment. Understanding what is going on during an attack is key, and learning simple exercises to regulate breathing and reduce anxiety can help people avoid further attacks, and to feel more in control.

What about Christians?!

One phrase is repeated hundreds of times across the Old and New Testaments: Do not be afraid/do not fear. It's clear that God's people struggle with anxiety just as much as anyone else. In fact, it's interesting to consider whether some Christians might be *more* at risk of anxiety, not because of their faith, but because of how it causes them to live. Great faith – and great passion (see 'Is your passion stressing you out?') changes how we live, meaning we push ourselves to new limits. As people seeking to grow in faith, and also in what we achieve for God, we often look to operate outside our comfort zones. God challenges us, moves us on and through God we can achieve things we never thought possible. But have you ever thought about what that means for your anxiety level? If anxiety is triggered by things which are uncertain, new or perhaps not guaranteed to be successful, we may find that operating *outside* our comfort zone means we are working very much *inside* our anxiety zone!

Here's an interesting quote, from a book called *Do No Harm*, by Henry Marsh. It is a memoir of the experiences of a neurosurgeon, and early in the opening chapters, he says this:

'...*as a surgeon you learn at an early stage of your career to accept intense anxiety as a normal part of the day's work and to carry on despite it.*'[2] Now I'm not comparing what we do for God to brain surgery (unless you are in fact a neurosurgeon!), but it may be a big change to think about anxiety in this way: as something that we will inevitably experience, but need to *manage.* Sometimes your brain may trigger anxiety, but the correct response is to carry on in spite of it. We need to learn how to manage anxiety well, to moderate and reduce it where we can, and perhaps harder for some of us, to *tolerate it* when we can't.

So what else does the Bible have to say about anxiety? There are two 'often quoted' passages in the New Testament that address the issue of anxiety and worry. It's really important to understand what they are actually saying, and that they are not offering trite, superficial advice, but good teaching. The first comes from the gospels and is recorded in Matthew 6 and Luke 12. Here Jesus advises us not to worry: 'about your life, what you will eat or drink; or about your body, what you will wear. Is not life more than food, and the body more than clothes? Look at the birds of the air; they do not sow or reap or store away in barns, and yet your heavenly Father feeds them. Are you not much more valuable than they? Can any one of you by worrying add a single hour to your life?' (Matthew 6:25-27, NIV). In short therefore, this passage reassures us that we don't need to worry because God has our needs covered. However, this standalone advice may be difficult to follow – and to understand. Clearly overcoming anxiety requires much more than just 'deciding' not to be anxious any more. But can the context of this passage shed some more helpful light on what is really needed in order to start to win back ground from anxiety?

This is yet another example of an often-quoted passage that starts with 'therefore'. If we just look at the words of verses 25-

---

2 Henry Marsh, *Do No Harm: Stories of Life, Death and Brain Surgery* (Weidenfeld and Nicolson, 2014).

27 we're missing the key point of what Jesus was saying. So what is it all about? The passage forms part of the famous Sermon on the Mount, and the key section that verses 25-27 flow out of is found in verses 19-24. Here Jesus concentrates on the conflicts that we might experience between the values of the world and God's values. It advises us to focus on storing 'treasures in heaven' rather than on earth (v. 20, NIV), and that 'You cannot serve both God and money' (v. 24).

Considering verses 25-27 in this context is interesting. It is this changed perspective, this managing to move away from what the world tells you is important, and looking instead at things through God's eyes and with God's perspective which leads on to the 'therefore, do not worry' section. This advice makes much more sense in terms of what this new understanding of life changes in terms of things you just don't need to worry about – clothes, food, these perhaps less vital aspects of life, become a lot less important if your focus is on heavenly things rather than the things our culture tells us are important. *The Message* puts it in its usual no nonsense way: 'If you decide for God, living a life of God-worship, it follows that you don't fuss about what's on the table at mealtimes or whether the clothes in your closet are in fashion. There is far more to your life than the food you put in your stomach, more to your outer appearance than the clothes you hang on your body. Look at the birds, free and unfettered, not tied down to a job description, careless in the care of God. And you count far more to him than birds' (Matthew 6:25-26, *The Message*). The antidote to some worry and anxiety is a change of perspective, a realisation of what is *really* important in life, so that a lot of our worries fade away. This is very similar advice to the things we considered in the chapter 'Wise building' – it is about what we build our lives upon and what therefore starts to be important. If we focus on God and place our trust in God a lot of our worries become less powerful.

By the way, that last verse of this passage is a great piece of advice. '*Can all your worries add a single moment to your life?*'

asks the NLT (Matthew 6:27). The futility of worrying is well worth considering – how much good does it ever do? I often encourage people instead of ruminating endlessly, to write down their worries on paper and try to work them through rationally – either to end with a decided action that they need to perform – or to decide to let it go. Getting thoughts out of your mind onto paper like this often helps put a stop to the endless cycle of worrying. Either decide to *do something about it* or decide to let it go!

So, what about the worries we have that persist in spite of this change of perspective? Paul's 'advice for life' chapter, in Philippians 4, has this to suggest: 'Don't fret or worry. Instead of worrying, pray. Let petitions and praises shape your worries into prayers, letting God know your concerns. Before you know it, a sense of God's wholeness, everything coming together for good, will come and settle you down. It's wonderful what happens when Christ displaces worry at the centre of your life.' (Phil 4:6-7, *The Message*). This is great advice for how to deal with worries that seize up our mind. Psalm 56:3 says: 'When I am afraid, I put my trust in you' (NIV), but Paul adds more to this, with specific advice about *how* to hand things over to God through prayer.

It's all very well being handed the advice to pray over the things that make us anxious – but is it good advice? Research would seem to suggest so, finding that those who regularly pray are in general less anxious and have lower stress levels. They also cope better with psychiatric treatment, which is a very stressful experience. People struggling with anxiety often feel they do not have very much control over their lives or the things they fear might happen. Prayer places our trust outside of ourselves, in God, who is much easier to place your faith in. The practice of prayer, with its similarities to some forms of mindfulness practice, may also help to calm anxiety and improve awareness of what is going on in your thoughts.

But Paul doesn't finish with his suggestion to pray. He has some further fantastic advice. If your mind is very active, and prone to rumination, it is very hard to just 'switch off' and stop thinking. This is particularly the case when you are anxious or stressed because part of the influence this state has on you is to make your mind particularly 'buzzing'. Did you know as well that your memory is automatically biased by your emotions? When you are feeling sad or anxious, your mind is much more likely to bring to the front of your memory times when you were feeling the same way. This all makes it so easy to get bogged down with sad or anxious thoughts in difficult times. Paul offers some great advice for those caught with very active minds – to focus them on good stuff instead. 'Finally brothers and sisters, whatever is true, whatever is noble, whatever is right, whatever is pure, whatever is lovely, whatever is admirable – if anything is excellent or praiseworthy – think about such things … and the God of peace will be with you' (Philippians 4:8–9, NIV).

If your mind is on fire and your thoughts are buzzing, channel them into something positive. If you cannot help but ruminate, focus on good things that trigger positive emotions and by doing so, start to smother the anxiety fires. This takes practice – don't give up if the first few times it is very hard. Be aware of your mind slipping back into the worries and gently but firmly pick yourself up and return to thinking about the good stuff! Mindfulness exercises can help with this, but you can also help yourself by making a scrapbook, or collecting a box full of things which remind you of positive things, happy memories, great things God has given you, good experiences – perhaps even good things about yourself if you are prone to getting bogged down with what feel like your failings. In those moments when worries overtake you, get the book/box out and deliberately spend some time wallowing in happy thoughts!

Fighting the fires of anxiety

Though the Bible holds some great advice, we've got to remember that it is rare for prayer *alone* to help if you are struggling with a significant anxiety problem. Do not feel bad about needing some further advice and support. Anxiety can feel terrifying, particularly because of the speed with which it can burst into flame. You may feel very out of control and this sense of having lost control of your own mind and body can add further anxiety to the mix and make things even worse. But be encouraged – fast as anxiety can come on, it can respond just as fast to good treatment and support. Once you understand your anxiety better, you will be able to start winning back ground and taking back control. So how do you begin to fight the fires of anxiety? Two things are important to realise from the start, and both are about things that commonly worry those struggling with anxiety.

Step One

The first is that the physical symptoms you are experiencing are most likely entirely related to the anxiety and not to any other underlying cause. Now, if you are experiencing specific worrying symptoms – chest pain, difficulty swallowing, persistent heartburn, headaches, dizziness, etc., you do need to get those checked out with your doctor. This is to rule out any other cause. But all of these can be caused by anxiety, and I have seen all improve dramatically once anxiety and stress levels are reduced following helpful treatment. Get them checked out rather than remaining gripped with worry over them. Note also that almost all the common symptoms of anxiety will produce a terrifying diagnosis if typed into Google! Take some good advice: *If you are struggling with anxiety do not turn to the internet!* Instead take them to your doctor and let him/her judge which need further investigations.

Once you have had the 'all clear' from your doctor, how do you manage the fact that the symptoms are still there? What you need to recognise is that they are *secondary* to – i.e. being caused by – the anxiety and stress. The best way to treat them is to treat the *anxiety and stress.* This will indirectly improve the symptoms. There are circumstances – when anxiety symptoms are interfering with your work or with exams for example, or if you have a big occasion coming up that you don't want your anxiety to affect – when your GP might be prepared to prescribe short term medications which block the effect of those anxiety hormones temporarily. However, these are a short term solution. Treating the underlying anxiety will be much more effective long-term than trying to treat the symptoms themselves.

Step Two

The second key thing to realise when fighting anxiety is that the thing you are dreading most – the WCS probably *won't happen.* Think for a moment about the Big Worries that have plagued you over recent years. How many actually did come true? Which was more damaging to your life in the end – the WCS (especially if it never happened) or the worry and anxiety you experienced? The experience of dread and fear is usually much worse than the actual reality.

Step Three

A key step in fighting anxiety – especially 'free floating' anxiety – is to reduce general stress levels as much as possible. Building regular relaxation into your life will help you to do this. Seek out things to do that are relaxing and try to fit at least one in every day. You may also want to learn a relaxation technique or exercise. This helps reduce stress in general the more you practice – but also once you have got used to it, your relaxation exercises can help to reduce anxiety levels *in the moment* if you are facing something you are afraid of. This gives you something to do when panic starts to set in, leaving you less vulnerable to anxiety and less 'at its mercy' when it strikes.[3] Remember though, learning a relaxation technique takes time, and the more you practise the better you will get. At first practise in times when you are feeling relatively calm anyway – do not jump in at the deep end and try a relaxation exercise when you are feeling really anxious! As you get more proficient at the exercise you'll find you can use it in less calm situations.

Step Four

As well as trying to dampen down the smouldering fires of anxiety, take a good look at what is fuelling them. Understanding and addressing thought patterns or values/goals you are living by which might be triggering a lot of anxiety is ultimately the key to reducing how often you have to deal with it. Specific fears or phobias can also be addressed very effectively by gradually stepping down those avoidance strategies, and learning good techniques to manage anxiety in the meantime. These are both part of the approach taken by cognitive behaviour therapy (CBT). There are lots of great resources that can help you to work through a CBT-based approach to anxiety. Why not think of working through one, whether alone or with a friend? Alternatively you may want to try to find a therapist to work with. Your GP may be able to refer you or recommend someone local, or you can find details of local therapists from one of the organisations listed in the resources section.

Be encouraged!

Anxiety can be really frightening, and can blow up incredibly fast. It can feel very powerful and out of control. But it holds all its power in the fact that because it is scary, you don't tend to challenge it. Once challenged a lot of the fear simply collapses

---

3   You can find a simple relaxation exercise in Appendix 2.

– like realising that a 'Beware of the Dog' sign is actually talking about a tiny fluffy poodle, its bark is worse than its bite! With good strategies and support, most people struggling with anxiety find they are able to win back control almost as quickly as it stole it from them in the first place. You may never be without anxiety – we all need to experience it to keep us safe. But you need not be at its mercy any more.

Over to you

How much would you agree with the following statement: I am a born worrier.

Not me at all   Totally true

On the whole would you say that for you, anxiety is helpful or unhelpful?

Are there any examples of things you have not done, or not wanted to do, because of anxiety?

How would your life be different if you experienced less anxiety?

Do you think any problems you have with anxiety are related to stress?

Have you ever experienced a panic attack? If so, write down what happened here …

Looking back, can you see how the anxiety triggered the physical symptoms?

How might this change the way you react if this happens again?

Do you regularly practice any kind of relaxation exercise? What difference might it make if you did? (Check out Appendix 2 for a simple relaxation exercise you could try!)

What do you think is your biggest challenge – to *reduce* your anxiety level, or learn to *manage* your anxiety better?

Thinking about the Big Worries that have preoccupied you over the last year or so – can you note any down you remember worrying about a lot? Which ones (if any) actually happened in the end?

It's easy to get bogged down in thinking about things that are negative, or worrying. Counteract that by deliberately thinking of things from Paul's list in Phil. 4:8-9 – things that are true, noble, right, pure, lovely, admirable, excellent, or praiseworthy. Can you note down some of these things? You might be able to find things to help you bring them to mind – photos, mementos, etc. Why not make a box of good things to help you in moments when you feel overwhelmed with worry?

14

Staying sane *long term*

Throughout this book we've been on a journey exploring the whole issue of stress, and developing a better understanding of where the stress in our own lives might be coming from. Stress really is everywhere, and very often the people most at risk are those with the most potential – people who are aiming high, working hard and striving to get the most out of their lives. Stress also hits you at particular times in your life – raising children being one classic example that almost guarantees to raise your stress levels, particularly if you juggle the demands of family life with a job.

So if you know you are struggling because of your personal stress level, what should your response be? I have already explained my frustration when people are told the 'correct' approach is simply to do less – to step down from some of the things they are trying to achieve and live a 'half-life' so that their ability to cope with stress is not exceeded. My experience is that people who take this advice often end up with more problems with stress rather than fewer – that their ability to cope with stress shrinks as the level of demands in their life falls. Once our confidence in our own ability to cope starts to become eaten away, stress becomes more and more an enemy that we fear.

A better approach to stress therefore needs to cover two angles. We need to know about how to deal with it right now

- particularly if it is triggering serious physical or emotional problems. But with stress all around us, we also need to learn how to handle it better *long term*. We need to develop our ability to cope with and manage stress. The more we are able to do this the more we will be able to achieve. I said right at the start of the book that many people I work with are more likely to be limited in their lives by their ability to handle stress than by other things such as ability or intelligence. The reverse is also true – if you look at people who have been successful in whatever their area, you tend to find that an ability to cope with stress and pressure well – to manage that pressure and avoid being crushed by it – is as important as how good they are at what they do. Their secret is something about learning how to stay sane in spite of the pressure; how to dampen the impact of the stress they experience and shake off its consequences.

Is it wrong to push the limits?

But before we go on and think about how to do this long term it is important to ask the question: Is it wrong to push the limits? This is particularly true from a biblical perspective – as we live in a world which increasingly moves further and further away from the biblical ideals of how to live. Our society is 24/7, high energy and high demand. Should we in fact be aiming to step away from that instead of learning how to cope with it better? I have heard many a sermon challenging the culture of busy-ness we live in – and with good reason. So do our *aims* need adjusting instead of our *brains*?!

To some degree this is a question we all need to ask ourselves very honestly. There are a whole host of areas where we have to make big decisions regarding where our priorities lie. Family or work, friends or career, church or social life – these are all everyday dilemmas for a lot of people. But deciding to make some things high priority does not mean that you cannot push the limits elsewhere. Instead deciding where those limits are and

defining some of the most important ones *enables* you to explore
what you can fit in to your time instead of reducing it.

The Bible is not a book for people who want to lie low, live
the quiet life. Instead it is full of messages which inspire us to
dream big, challenge ourselves, fit the most in. Isaiah 45 gives
this advice when thinking about the future and what God might
do through you: 'Enlarge the place of your tent, stretch your tent
curtains wide, do not hold back' (v. 2, NIV). We have explored in
this book where some of our passions and drives might cause us
to slip up where stress is concerned – but that doesn't mean we
should aim to no longer have those passions. Instead the verse
goes on to give good advice about how to sustain and support
this striving: 'lengthen your cords, strengthen your stakes'. The
instinct to push the limits is a good, often God-driven one,
as is the energy and drive to achieve big things for God. But
we mustn't forget the just as important call to strengthen our
safety ropes and secure our anchors to the things that keep us
grounded in tough, busy times.

If you want to push the limits, you need to be *really* good
at managing stress. You must not neglect this area of your life.
It supports and enables the other things. Carry on pushing the
limits without sorting this out and eventually you will risk
falling flat on your face.

So here are a few tips for how to successfully push the limits
and keep your sanity:

1 - Draw some sensible lines

I know that you want to say yes to everything people ask you
to do. I know that you want to 'have it all'. But remember that
you cannot escape being human. Draw some sensible lines, agree
some basic limits to what you do. Do not forget the parts of
your life which are a lot less negotiable. If you do not leave a
bit of flexibility in your life, when those things (e.g. children)
suddenly need more time for whatever reason (illness, crises,

being teenagers) you risk being pushed over your capacity to cope.

If possible, agree some of these basic lines with the input of the people who need you the most. Think about things like how many evenings/weekends it is *reasonable* to be 'booked up' on; how much time on an average day you *actually* have to work on reports/planning/baking/whatever it is you are prone to volunteering for; how long it *realistically* takes to write something/direct the Christmas play/mentor that person, etc. Think about your basic needs and make sure you have time for them: for sleep especially. Research recently released revealed that one of the biggest causes of insufficient sleep is not actually insomnia, but people procrastinating (i.e. getting side-tracked into doing other things!) when they should be going to bed. I know you won't stick to it every night but think about how much sleep you need, what time you have to get up - and do the maths! You certainly won't sleep if you are sitting up watching *Newsnight* or cutting out stars for next Sunday's children's church when you should be in bed!

Included amongst your list should be some 'non-negotiables'. These are things that you set into your life schedule which are there in order to make sure you can maintain the pace without running out of steam. They must be as set in stone as it is possible for them to be. Here are some things I suggest you consider making non-negotiables (ignore those which do not apply to your situation):

- Not working past a certain hour in the evenings (except in *genuine* emergency situations)
- Turning your work email *off* at weekends/at the end of the working day
- Not taking work calls outside of work hours (again, except in *genuine* emergencies)
- Scheduling at least 30 minutes each day of uninterrupted 'you' time.
- Taking all the holiday time you are entitled to at work.

- Actually fitting in at least half of any time 'in lieu' you are due at work.
- Always accepting, and arranging times when someone offers to babysit.
- Reading at least one book each month which has nothing to do with work.
- Spending regular time each week with God, in prayer and reading your Bible.
- Fitting in at least three slots of genuine relaxation into each week.
- Making at least one a time each month where you get away from the house, work, etc., and into the outdoors.

These things are by definition not easy to put into your life. Very few things worth doing are! There will always be the temptation to push them out again. Remember why they are there! They could be the most important things in your week – not the things that *stop* you from working efficiently but the things that *enable* you to work efficiently and fit so much in.

2 - Change your attitude!

So now I am going to say something that you might feel is surprising – we need to stop seeing stress as the enemy. I know – all of this book has been about looking at the impact stress can have on us, and the reasons it is BAD for us. But do you know something? Research into which people have the biggest negative impact from stress demonstrates that it is more to do with how you view stress than how much you experience. People who see stress as a bad thing and view it as the enemy are much more likely to experience negative consequences from the stress that they experience.

So here's some bad news: stress is inevitable, and you are going to experience some high stress moments in your life. But here is the good news – it needn't destroy you. Stress is, after all, designed to improve your performance. Recognise it for what it is, use it in positive ways and, most importantly of all, take care of how you react to it so that you do not make things worse rather than better, and stress needn't be your enemy.

It's very important that we change our attitude towards stress and stop thinking with a 'victim mentality' about it. Instead of just sitting back and letting stress waves break over our head, we can take control and modify our own experiences of stress. Next time you walk into a storm, remind yourself that you are in control! Do not let your emotional smoke alarms have you immediately running for cover: take some deep breaths and think about what is triggering them. Think about looking into the way that approaches like CBT can change the way you think and make you much better at dealing with stress. Use some of the approaches and ideas suggested in this book to put yourself in a better position to manage stress and you might be surprised by how much your own experience of it changes.

3 - Get into good routines

Think about some routines that are about what you *do* rather than what you *don't do* as well. We are all used to the idea of doing things in order to preserve our physical health – trying to eat 5-a-day, do a bit of exercise each week, etc. Why are we so bad at doing the same for our *emotional* health? Make some plans and stick to them! These are things that you need to include in your week – which are just as important *if not more so* than the things that usually eat up your time. We need a total mind shift in how we view our priorities! Time out to relax, or catch up with friends, or get into the countryside must not be just something you do when you have nothing else to do – it needs to be something you schedule. If you don't you will hardly ever fit it in.

Here then lies some interesting advice for staying sane long term. Do push the limits in terms of what you aim to fit in, but this is an important truth: **if you cannot fit in time to keep yourself emotionally and physically healthy, you are doing too much**. Push the limits, don't pretend there are none.

4 - Recognise early warning signs

This is another area where your 'nearest and dearest' can help. How well do you know the early warning signs that you are getting stressed out? How do you know when your stress baseline has started to rise above the comfort zone? Learn to recognise and become aware of the little things you do as your stress level starts to rise. The principle here is very similar to that described for managing anger. The sooner you intervene to manage stress or deal with problems, the easier it will be. Your aim in managing stress long term should be to try not to let it rise beyond the point where it starts to impact your life.

So, what are your personal warning signs? These may be physical (e.g. headaches, trouble sleeping); emotional (feeling tearful or irritable); practical (e.g. realising you have not had time to do certain things in a long while); or social (losing touch with people whose support and friendship you really value, or not having the energy to connect with them). Have a think about what you think yours might be – and then discuss them with the people who know you best. You might be surprised what they notice and you do not.

Once you have a better idea of what your personal 'signs and symptoms' of stress might be, you can note down some early warning signs for yourself. It may be that you cannot change the stress you are under straight away – but your being aware of it will help, and enable you to build in more stress management strategies to get you through that particular stormy patch. Most of all it will avoid the risk of you running headlong into burnout without realising that it is just around the corner.

5 - Get some perspective

We've talked a lot in this book about pushing the limits - fitting in the most you can and getting the best out of life. Passion is a good thing - something that drives and motivates this desire to do as much as possible. We must be really careful that we don't slip into any other motivation. Most of all we must not become taken in by our culture, which tells us that we are what we achieve and that our value lies in what we do. We must keep our eyes seeing our lives from God's perspective.

I have always thought that one of the most interesting people in the Bible is Enoch. He doesn't get a lot of page space. In fact everything that is said about him can be fitted into a few lines – a couple of verses in Genesis and then a couple more in Hebrews. Enoch was one of the descendants of Adam through Seth. He's included in the list in Genesis 5: 'Enoch lived 365 years, walking in close fellowship with God. Then one day he disappeared, because God took him' (vv. 23-23, NLT). What is interesting about Enoch is that this is all Genesis tells us about him - yet he appears in Hebrews 11 in a list of Old Testament characters of note because of their amazing faith (Hebrews 11:5-6). Enoch appears alongside people like Abraham and Noah - people who have chapters of the Old Testament telling their story. All we know about him was that he had great faith – and that because of this God took him to be with him. It is easy to get bogged down in debate over whether he never actually died or not - but what interests me is that what we're told is *enough*. What is important to God is not our acts, what we achieve or the great stuff we pack into life, but that we follow God faithfully. Hebrews tells us Enoch '*was known as a person who pleased God*' (Hebrews 11:5 NLT). That is God's perspective on what matters in our lives. So much as we are passionate, much as we desire to achieve things for God, much as we long to change things for the better here, tell people about God or help them get to know God better, the thing that really matters is that we place our faith and trust in God. Anything and everything that we do or achieve comes second to this.

Our attitude to stress must be one of treating it with respect – because it can have a big impact on us and our ability to do what God calls us to do. But at the same time we must put it in perspective. God's love is bigger, and it is our faith in God that gives us the confidence we need to be able to weather periods of stress. As Paul says in Romans 8, 'Do you think anyone is going to be able to drive a wedge between us and Christ's love for us? There is no way! Not trouble, not hard times, not hatred, not hunger, not homelessness, not bullying threats, not backstabbing, not even the worst sins listed in Scripture … None of this fazes us because Jesus loves us. I'm absolutely convinced that nothing – nothing living or dead, angelic or demonic, today or tomorrow, high or low, thinkable or unthinkable – absolutely nothing can get between us and God's love because of the way that Jesus our Master has embraced us' (Romans 8:35-39, *The Message*).

This then – this ultimate foundation on the rock of God's love an acceptance, not for what we do but for who we are, must be our greatest defence against stress. Because at the end of the day if we achieve nothing in life but being ourselves, that is enough for God.

6 - Superheroes never work alone

Early on in this book I broke the perhaps sad news that whoever you are, you are most likely 'just' human. But there's nothing wrong with wanting to achieve super-hero like things for God! Remember, however, that superheroes never work on their own. Here are some key people you might need to include in your stress management plan.

Your doctor

In this book we've touched on some fairly significant health matters – physically and emotionally. This may have brought to mind things that you need to discuss with your Doctor. Do! This may not be easy, and it may require some planning – but it is important. Do not put off getting things checked out if you need to. This book is no replacement for good, personal medical advice from someone who has seen and knows you personally.

Sailed into a storm? An aside on medication
A common question I am asked by those struggling with stress is whether or not they should take medication. Most people are reluctant to – and it is rarely the answer *on its own*. But as part of a combined set of approaches designed to help you learn better strategies for dealing with stress, it can have a very good place. This is particularly the case if life is hurling a majorly stressful situation at you right at the moment. This will not last forever, and while it is there you may find that some medication helps you to stay on top of things until they calm down. In particular, medication can help reduce that all-too- troublesome rumination and help bring down the ferocity of obsessive thought patterns.

Here's my favourite analogy to explain the role of medication in treating stress related emotional problems like anxiety and depression. Imagine that life is about sailing a boat across the sea. Every now and then you sail into some rough water, and waves come over the side of the boat. So, you have to bail water out. Usually this is no problem at all, but if you sail into a really big storm then you might find that all the bailing becomes exhausting, that you are unable to do much else *except* bail, or that in spite of your bailing the water levels are rising and you fear you might go under. In addition to the storms we might encounter in life, many of us find that for whatever reason – be it childhood experiences, personality factors or other things entirely - our boats also are not entirely water-tight. They leak, or even have holes that need patching up. These holes may not be so noticeable in everyday life because we can easily bail enough to keep afloat. But once we sail into a storm they can become really problematic. Now, taking medication doesn't seal those holes, which, in the long term, is probably what we need to do in order to improve our resilience to stress. But what it does do is a bit like dropping in someone else to help bail. It makes things slightly easier, and often that can give us the headspace and breathing space we need to get down to doing some longer-term repairs on those holes or leaking points. And if the storm is unusually heavy, medication can get us through the roughest times - and once things calm again we can return to normal and gradually stop taking it.

Your friends

I know part of being a superhero is that smouldering isolation, the things that make you so different from other people that they keep you apart. But the truth is, we are all human and we all experience stress! In general we'd all be a lot better off if we all shared more of it. Do not hide your worries from your friends. But do not just use them to moan at either! Take time to share, bounce ideas around, suggest solutions, and help each other see things in perspective.

In Genesis 2:28, God says this: 'It is not good for the man to be alone' (NIV). Did you know you were created to be in community? All humans were created in the image of God, and at the core of God is this wonderful mysterious community. In those early words of God's recorded in the Bible, we see that even the work of creation was a shared thing; God says, 'let *us* make mankind in *our* image' (Genesis 1:28, NIV). Something basic and vital at your very core reaches out to other humans. That is why loneliness is such a huge issue - and why it has deep reaching effects on our physical and emotional health. We cannot flourish if we are disconnected from other humans. So rejoice in those connections. Make a deliberate effort to make time to nurture them.

Someone you can be 'accountable' to

This chapter asks you to make some key, clear decisions about things you aim to change. You may well have other notes from other chapters with actions you need to take. Once you have decided on these things, think about making yourself accountable to someone else. You are much more likely to stick to them if you share them.

Why not find a friend or colleague with whom you can be honest – even better if they also want to improve how they manage stress. Aim to agree three things you are going to try to stick to for the next month to see how it improves your stress levels. Then agree to meet up weekly or fortnightly to chat about how it is going. And once the month is up, adjust your lines if you need to, and commit to three things for the next three months. Keep meeting up; follow the advice of 1 Thessalonians 5:11: 'encourage one another and build each other up' (NIV).

Whatever you do ...

This book has covered a wide variety of topics and perspectives. And the people who read it will bring a similarly wide variety of experiences with them. We all experience stress in different ways. We all respond to it in different ways. And it affects us all in different ways. The point of this book is not to somehow *avoid* stress. In fact it is the opposite – it is to recognise it as part of our essential experience of being human. Our limits are not limitations – they are part of the way we were created, and an echo of the God who created us.

Perhaps that is the key to how we manage stress – that ultimate perspective setter. As Paul puts it so well in Colossians,

'Whatever you do, work at it with all your heart, as working for the Lord, not for human masters, since you know that you will receive an inheritance from the Lord as a reward. It is the Lord Christ you are serving' (Col. 3:23-24, NIV).

We are not called to 'skimp or trim' in our time upon this earth. We are not inspired to live cautious, held back lives. We are called to push the limits. But we've got to be careful about why we do this. Do not do it to feel worthwhile, to build your self-esteem, to prove other people right or wrong. Do it for God and for this reason alone.

Because we work for God, because it is so important to us, because we are so passionate, be careful to work within a structure that protects you from your own limits. If stress has forced you to stop, do not feel bad for yearning to get going again. But do put in sensible limits to help you stay on top of stress. Learning to manage stress and stopping it from holding you back will leave you free-er in the long run. So do work with all your heart. Push on, dream big and aim high!

Just never ever forget you are human.

Over to you ...

Are there areas in your life where you are aware of 'pushing the limits'?

Have you ever pushed it too far?

Are there any changes you need to make in order to remain within your own human limits?

1 - Draw some sensible lines

Here are the suggested non-negotiables you might need to think about. Tick any you think should be non-negotiable in YOUR life. Are there any you want to add?

- Not working past a certain hour in the evenings (except in GENUINE emergency situations).
- Turning your work email OFF at weekends/at the end of the working day.
- Not taking work calls outside of work hours (again, except in GENUINE emergencies).
- Scheduling at least 30 minutes each day of uninterrupted 'you' time.
- Taking all the holiday time you are entitled to at work.
- Actually fitting in at least half of any time 'in lieu' you are due at work.
- Always accepting, and arranging times when someone offers to babysit.
- Reading at least one book each month which has nothing to do with work.
- Spending regular time each week with God, in prayer and reading your Bible.
- Fitting at least three slots of genuine relaxation into each week.
- Make at least one a time each month where you get away from the house, work, etc. and into the outdoors.

2 - Good routines

What are some good, healthy routines that you want to prioritise in your life? Think about the 4 key areas which tend to get impacted by stress:

EMOTIONAL

PHYSICAL

PRACTICAL

SOCIAL

Are there any changes you need to make NOW in order to fit more of these key things into your life?

3 - Recognise early warning signs

Imagine your personal signs and symptoms of stress are a bit like a traffic light. They give you an indication of what action you might need to take. Have a go at filling in the following diagram - what do these three levels feel like, and how should you respond to each?

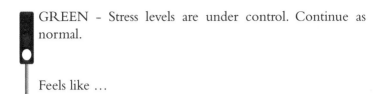

GREEN - Stress levels are under control. Continue as normal.

Feels like …

Actions to take?

AMBER - Stress levels are at warning stage. Be aware and take action to avoid problems.

Feels like …

Actions to take?

RED - Stress levels approaching burnout. Need to STOP.

Feels like …

Actions to take?

4 – Get some perspective.

Think about the things that have stressed you out over the last month or so. See if you can write down as many as you can remember.

How many of these will matter in …
… a month?
… a year?
… a lifetime?

If you think about the things that please God, and are about following God, how might that change your priorities?

5 - Superheroes never work alone

Thinking about this book as a whole, are there any issues it has raised that you need to discuss with your GP?

If you are going to be successful - particularly long term - at achieving and maintaining the changes you have noted throughout this book, the single most important thing you can do is to make yourself accountable to someone. Make a plan to meet with that person, chat this through (Why not get them a copy of the book too!) and tell them three things you want to change *now* (you can add more in future months!).

Be specific in your plans of things to change. Do not just write 'work less': write down clear goals, e.g. 'I will not work beyond 7 pm on weekdays or at weekends unless it is a genuine emergency. I will note down any actions I think of in those times on my phone to remind me to do them the next working day.'

Person you are going to be accountable to:

Plans for first meeting:

Your three SPECIFIC things you commit to do/change:

1

2

3

Appendix 1: Links for further support and information

For **general support, resources and information surrounding mental health issues, and specific issues affecting the church** go to **Mind and Soul** (www.mindandsoul.info) – a national organisation encouraging the church to engage in issues relating to emotional and mental health. Mind and Soul also has links to other organisations who can offer support related to specific mental health problems.

For **information about how the church can engage more effectively** with those struggling with emotional and mental health problems, including those associated with stress and burnout, check out the **Mental Health Access Pack** (www.mentalhealthaccesspack.org).

For **someone to talk to/advice and prayer Premier Lifeline** (http://www.premier.org.uk/Premier-Lifeline/About-Premier-Lifeline) offers confidential support. Call 0300 111 0101 from 9am-midnight every day of the year.

For **advice with specific mental health issues**:

Eating disorders: Anorexia and Bulimia Care (www. anorexiabulimiacare.org.uk) is the national Christian organisation supporting all those struggling with eating disorders. They have a specific helpline for sufferers (03000 11 12 13 then option 2), and another for the parents of teens and younger children (03000 11 12 13 then option 1).

Self-harm: selfharmUK (selfharm.co.uk/home) is a national organisation providing support and resources about self-harm. They also run an online program called Alumina for teens aged 14-18 who are struggling with self-harm (http://alumina. selfharm.co.uk)

Secular organisations/websites

MIND (www.mind.org.uk) is a secular mental health charity, providing information and support relating to all mental health problems.

YoungMINDS (www.youngminds.org.uk) focuses on mental health problems in children and young people and offers excellent advice for parents as well as a great website for children and teens.

The Samaritans (http://www.samaritans.org/how-we-can-help-you/contact-us) are a secular organisation offering support for anyone struggling with emotional or mental health issues. Call them any time, any day, on 08457 90 90 90, email jo@ samaritans.org write to them at Freepost RSRB-KKBY-CYJK, Chris, PO Box 90 90, Stirling, FK8 2SA or follow links to find your local branch.

Appendix 2: A simple relaxation exercise

If you want a really simple relaxation exercise to try, here's one to give a go. Select a song that you like and find calms you, or helps you feel more in control and positive. Very often people find that worship songs work really well here, but you might want to go for something else. Make sure it is a song you really like, though, as you'll be listening to it quite a bit!

Put the song on – if you can (on an mp3 player/cd player), put it on repeat. Get yourself comfortable – it doesn't matter whether you are sitting or lying down, eyes open or closed, on the floor or on a chair, do whatever feels most relaxing to you. You may want to make the room or space relaxing too – think dimming the lights, make sure you are nice and warm, maybe light a candle. Listen to the song, and as you listen, either sing or hum along with the tune or phrases. This might feel like a slightly mad thing to do, but it really helps to regulate your breathing. Here's also where worship or Christian songs can be great because singing along with the words also helps you to connect with God and with what the song is reminding you.

Repeat this two or three times – right through the song. You can use more than one song if you like – this can be a really relaxing thing to do. But using one song over and over again will help you start to associate that song with being relaxed, making it easier to calm yourself each time you hear it. Repeat this exercise several times a week, at times when things are calm. Remember to hum or sing the song quietly as you rest. Focus on the words or tune, how it feels as you hum, and the sense of calmness as you sing.

After a while, as well as relaxing in the moments when you practice this exercise, you will find that it becomes something you can practice in stressful moments when out and about. Some people keep the song with them on an mp3 or on their phone so they can actually listen to it, but you may find that just humming it through quietly or even letting it play in your mind helps. If you hit a stress attack, grab a few minutes to be by yourself – a quiet corridor works, or nip to the loo. Then use that time to focus on the song and again hum through; or if you don't want to be overheard, just hum it silently. The calming of your breathing will really help you to relax in the moment.

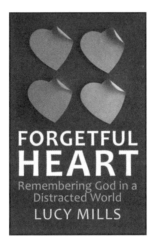

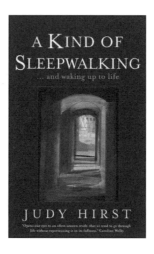

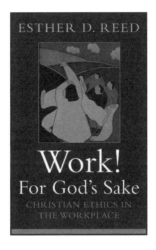

DARTON·LONGMAN✝TODD

PICK ME UP RANGE
Winner - BMA Popular Medicine Book 2013

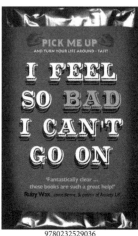

9780232529036

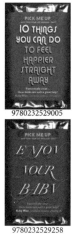

9780232529005

9780232529258

'Fantastically clear…these books are such a great help!'
Ruby Wax, comedienne and patron of Anxiety UK

These amazing little books are potential life-savers. Using simple text and bold design, each book meets the reader at a point of low mood or unhelpful thinking, and guides them through rational thought processes to a more positive mood and a healthier outlook on life.